Hardwired to Heal...

What if your body held the magic to heal itself and your illness was optional?

Vicki Ariatti

Hardwired to Heal is a commonsense guide to Natural Healing. Numerous golden concepts and principles are sprinkled like gold dust on each page that are clues for you as you ponder your own answers and solutions to put you on a healing trajectory that can make what seems "impossible" possible with natural healing. These golden nuggets will also highlight methods of how to work with your own innate healing power.

www.VickisWellness.com

Copyright © 2020 All rights reserved.

Hardwired to Heal...What if your body held the magic to heal itself and your illness was optional?

ISBN: 978-0-578-65730-1

PREFACE

When I was 8 years old, I made a vow that when I grew up, I was going to save children from childhood abuse and neglect. I thought I was going to be a nurse. As a teenager I switched my career to be a social worker. Little did I know that I would ease into naturopathic medicine.

Most people know me as the therapist with "magic hands". I have helped well over 700 people who kept searching for relief despite numerous disappointments. This has made me ponder what sets me apart from other therapists who don't get the same results and why their clients come to me.

My special gift is the ability to read your energy while listening to your body tell me specifically what it needs. That becomes your protocol for that treatment while resolving the particular pain point and imbalance while making corrections

I'm living my childhood vow and dream of making a difference to those who suffer. I simply combine my Gift of Healing, classroom education and intuition into unique signature protocols tailored for each individual client.

Holistic Energy Healing blesses the lives of my clients in ways that seem like magic. There is no magic or woo woo. I simply work with Energy,

Biology, Physiology and Anatomy, which is already hardwired by God for natural self-healing.

Hardwired to Heal is all about how your body is hardwired to heal itself and how you can assist in your own healing. This educational material is intended to give you hope, encouragement and tools so that you too can regain your wellness and live your life to its fullest on your terms.

Table of Contents

INTRODUCTION

Growing up without my mother left a big hole in my soul. Oh, how I longed for my mother's love. I remember the day I really thought we were all going to be together for good. Mom had found us a "beautiful" house with a fireplace, spacious bedrooms and a large family area.

To my surprise we all moved into this filthy roach infested nasty house with a strange man I had never seen before. It was a house I was willing to tolerate just to be with my mother. As a twelve-year-old I was finally going to be able to be a kid and give back the role of mother to my mother for my two younger sisters! Three days later our mother moved out.

The strange man stayed with us. We were clear across town in a neighborhood I had never been in before. There we were, stuck!

We didn't have cell phones back in 1963. We

didn't have a phone in this house. I was scared. I just wanted my mother but she didn't want me. My emotions were all over the place. I cried myself to sleep at night longing for my mother.

The man she left us with began to comfort me. He comforted me in a very inappropriate way. He made me feel safe and loved. I was special to him. He taught me how to have satisfying love. It felt like I was his wife. He took good care of me. I had a temporary boost in my self-esteem. I was a "somebody" to him who was lovable for the first time in my life. I truly felt special.

After a couple of months my sisters went back home to live with our step-dad. I refused to go. I was tired of being home alone and having to take care of my little sisters. Don't get me wrong, I loved my sisters, but I wanted someone to take care of me.

Doc moved me into his house with his pregnant wife and kids. Doc made me feel special and loved. His wife accepted me. His kids were like my little brothers and sisters. I finally had a family until my Aunt found out that I was being preyed upon by a pedophile.

My Aunt Mechling called Social Services and I was jerked out of my comfortable home while the search for Doc ensued. "Where are you taking me?" I asked the social workers. "Back to your mom's house", he replied. "Oh no you're not!" I demanded. "If you take me back there, I'll run away and no one will ever find me", I insisted! "They don't love me and I'm tired of being neglected!" I said as I put my foot down.

He looked at his partner and said, "What are we going to do with this child"? He kept driving. They whispered. We ended up in downtown Jackson, Mississippi.

My head was spinning. Where is he taking me?", I thought. We pulled up to the city jail. Oh my gosh! Was I being arrested for refusing to go back home? I was escorted to a jail cell with no explanation. As the metal door closed I felt like a prisoner. I went from a loving home to jail. Here I was left to wonder what I did that was so bad to be locked up like a criminal.

I was ashamed of myself for even being alive. As the hours ticked into days with no visitors, no change of clothes and no deodorant I began to stink.

Then magic happened midway through that week. I had a visitor, a female social worker came to visit me. She took me outside in the fresh air for a long walk. I felt like someone really cared about me.

I was so depressed, locked up in a cage like a wild animal with no one to talk to. I hated getting my plate of food through the bars in the steel door. Breathing fresh air and soaking up the sunshine felt so good. For that moment I didn't feel like a criminal. She informed me that they found my dad and he was going to come and get me and my little sisters. I felt relief until the metal doors closed behind me again.

Hours turned back into days waiting for my dad to come. I slipped into a very deep depression and wanted to die. I willed myself death to the point that I slept for 23 hours. I was so angry that I woke up that I said out loud, "Ok, if I'm going to live then I'm going to be a somebody." My vow as an 8-year-old to end childhood abuse and neglect took on even more meaning four years later. Kids should not be treated like this.

At the end of that long and dreadful week the social worker did come back and pick me up. She took me to my grandmother's house. It felt so good to be out of jail. It felt so good to take a shower and put on clean clothes. I once again was reunited with my sisters as we waited at our grandmother's house for our dad.

As years merged into decades my dream of being a "somebody" and my vow as an 8-year-old of saving kids from abuse and neglect got buried under "life". Who was I to think that I could change the world anyway?

After I married the second time, I got caught up in a downward spiral of unhealthy food choices since my new husband didn't like to eat healthy foods. I went along to get along not realizing that I was in a self-defeating mindset of not caring about me and my body AGAIN. I just gave into his food choices to avoid making two separate meals three times a day while slipping easily back into my old eating habits. I didn't have a mirror, so I didn't realize that I was packing on the pounds. Pounds that were ugly, unhealthy and self-destructive.

Biscuits and gravy didn't give my body the nourishment it needed and just made me hungrier. I loved homemade chocolate chip cookies and would sit with a bucket of vanilla ice cream and eat until I had brain freeze. I made homemade bread and would drown slice after slice in butter and gorge until the loaf finally cooled off before I quit eating it.

I was always hungry because my body wasn't getting the nourishment, it craved from real food. I worked my way up to a whopping 302 pounds. Arthritis, Sleep Apnea, Type 2 Diabetes and depression became crippling companions. I kept this weight on for SIX years. Then...

A television ad caught my attention as my brain swirled with possibilities. A local pharmacy was hosting a weight loss competition. "What if I could win some money", I thought as I argued with myself. I vacillated with whether the effort would be worth it. I wrestled with the possibilities.

"How can you save the world when you're not motivated to even save yourself?", I reasoned. I decided to step out of my comfort zone, put my big girl panties on and be a somebody just like I vowed when I was an eight-year-old little girl.

During the first weight loss competition in January 2010, I met Nancy Gossi who was my food coach. She gave me amazing supplements that really turned my health around. Her coaching taught me a lot about food and set me on a much better healing trajectory.

Unfortunately, I didn't address the emotional aspects of yo-yo dieting and eventually regained almost all that I had lost. I didn't address this aspect until the second weight loss challenge. This is when I began peeling back the layers of traumas and self-healing which sparked my love for Naturopathic Medicine and Energy Healing.

I was introduced to Energy Healing with Tracy which sparked my love of natural healing. I wanted to be like Tracy when I grew up. I chuckled with myself as Tracy was in her 30's and I was already 58.

Fortunately, it wasn't long before I was introduced to classes where I studied how emotions directly affect us physically while learning various methods of clearing and releasing those emotions. We studied homeopathy and learned to make homeopathic medicine. We received a working knowledge of essential oils and herbs.

During this classroom training we studied

Applied Acupressure as we broke out in groups and practiced on each other for our personal healing. This class led to a Cranial Sacral Therapy class, massage school and numerous other healing modality classes.

My personal journey of healing and energy healing classes guided me to become a therapist. I have a unique advantage over therapists who receive no more than classroom instruction in bodywork. I have been given the gift of being able to "listen" to my client's bodies and assist them in healing. I have learned to read energy and understand its unspoken language.

While overcoming my own traumas, pain and dysfunction I developed a true and lasting compassion for my fellow man. Out of adversity was born my "can do" attitude that my grandmother Sara instilled in me as a very young child. I'm a product of what I now offer to you.

My clients relate to me on a much deeper level of trust as I transfer hope, confidence and my "can do" attitude into their treatments. They know that I will do everything possible to make "impossible possible". My "job" is truly more of a mission.

This book is an introduction to what I have learned about the body's innate ability to heal itself. I'm going to teach you methods and modalities that are proven to work. This book is an introduction and overview of how your body is hardwired to heal itself.

These modalities and methods will be detailed in my online and offline classes so that you can help yourself, your family members and perhaps your own clients one day.

Those of you looking for alternatives to commercialized medicine will glean easy to understand and helpful techniques which will assist you in your wellness journey.

ACKNOWLEDGEMENT

Thank you to my mother for giving me life and not being able to be there for me. I love you. I know you were sick. Growing up as an independent take charge go-getter out of necessity has given me the foundation for my career today.

I'm grateful to my bonus dad Johnny who really is my dad and my grandmother Sara who did the best they could under the overwhelming circumstances. I appreciate your wisdom and examples. I love you.

Thank you to my children, Donna, Donald, Donovan, Billy and Jeffrey. I love you. Thank you for teaching me how to be a mother as I struggled while practicing on you. It would have been much easier if I knew what I was doing. For realz.

Thank you for the beautiful grandchildren you gave me who allowed me a second chance as a parent. I appreciate your children and your children's children as I experience parenthood and childhood through them. It's a joy to watch you grow and raise beautiful children of your own.

Thank you to my special friends, Hardy and June Anderson who were the first to guide me into my healing journey. It's no telling where I would be today without your friendship, long suffering, guidance and influences that are still with me today. I certainly didn't have what it took to put up with me during my transformation of messy mess metamorphosis of healing my little girl. I love and appreciate you.

Thank you, Suzanne Evans and your Driven Business School staff, for my extended business education that has set me on a trajectory for "Being Seen" as a professional.

Thank you, Vickie Gould and your expertise, in coaching, teaching and writing bestsellers. My dream of sharing my story of triumph over disaster and turning my talent, expertise and gift of healing into a book and course material is truly a dream come true.

Thank you, Nancy Gossi and Nat and Silence Weeks who are also instrumental in, directing me on my healing trajectory as food and nutrition coaches.

Thank you, LaRee Westover and my class, members. I did some serious healing my little girl in your Chrysalis classes learning energy healing. I use the valuable education, intuition and various modalities that I learned in my sessions with clients. This holistic approach to wellness is what sets me apart from other therapists in my field so that my clients experience healing in the way their body asks.

CHAPTER 1:   Let Food Be Your Medicine

"Let food be thy medicine and medicine be thy food."
Hippocrates

"All we need for health and healing has been provided by God in Nature... the challenge of Science is to find it.."
Paracelsus 16th Century A.D.

When I met my second husband, he was on three prescription drugs, two for pain and another one for depression that he called his "nut" pill. He lived to eat. He ate for taste not health.

He wasn't interested in his health if it meant changing his diet. He was a meat and potatoes man who loved his pies, donuts and cobblers for dessert.

His idea of a healthy breakfast was biscuits and sausage gravy.

Before I met Bill I was building muscle and burning off fat. I was toned and strong. Unfortunately, when we got married, I didn't stick to my own health food choices. I joined him in eating unhealthy again. I knew better but it seemed easier than making two separate meals three times a day. I just didn't think about my yo-yo ride to getting fat again.

"Here we go again! You wanna take another ride?", my body seemed to say. My muscled, toned and healthy body was just a fleeting moment as I packed on a whopping eighty five pounds the first ten months we were married.

I was three hundred and two pounds before I quit growing. I was so miserable that I couldn't move and breathe at the same time. I felt sick all the time. I didn't realize at the time that this was a subconscious pattern of self-abuse. I realized later that the emotional aspect of my vacillating health was my way of not loving myself.

I developed sleep apnea and ran a chain saw all night. I seriously don't know how he got any sleep. I went to bed exhausted and woke up tired. My joints ached with Arthritis and my blood sugar test strip gave me a frowning face when it showed me a reading of one hundred and twenty-six. That was high for me.

It took watching an ad on television SIX times about a local $10,000 weight loss challenge before I worked up the motivation to join. I was comfortable after losing 20 pounds on my own and was not motivated to do anything else. That 20 pounds made it easier to breathe and I really was comfortable being uncomfortable.

In fact, motivating myself to get up and make changes was extremely painful. I had to force myself after the first month by thinking about the prize money. I didn't change my "why" to wanting to be healthy for two years.

One of the vendor food coaches during the first challenge gave me a packet of information about eating low glycemic fruits and vegetables and incorporating a small percentage of proteins. She also gave me a monthly supply of nutraceuticals for five months to help me through.

The only exercise I could do was walk and ride

my bike. Cardio exercises and working out in the gym was so painful because my heart was weak and my body was heavy and out of shape. I was allergic to pain. I was too comfortable being uncomfortable and getting stronger was work. The thought of winning prize money was very appealing and kept me going.

Bill continued to eat his junk food and continued his downward spiral while I was busy repairing my health and getting well. By this time, he was up to twelve prescription drugs.

We were playing "see saw" with our health. Little did I know about the emotional aspect of yo yo dieting. I only focused on the physical aspect not realizing that I was beginning my journey into the world of holistic energy healing and epigenetics with my own wellness journey.

I was heading into a new world while he held steadfast to his motto: "I'd rather die happy eating what I want rather than eat the crap you eat. I'm not a rabbit," he touted.

We soon figured out that his headaches were due to high blood pressure. His lungs were also damaged by a couple of rounds of pneumonia. He used oxygen and an inhaler to breathe.

He had a heart arrhythmia that he had as far back as he could remember as an adult. His dad also had the same arrhythmia. When his heart skipped a couple of beats it mimicked a heart attack and would lay him out flat for a few hours like a limp dishrag.

Trying to stabilize him was a full time job until...his body pulled out a can of "whoop ass" on him to get his attention. He was dying in misery.

Inflammation created pain throughout his whole body. He was weak. His brain fog was so bad that he couldn't remember where he put things. I'm sure you know what I mean by putting something in a safe place and then losing the safe place?

Mental confusion moved in and overpowered his functioning brain cells. Arthritis was ripping the mobility out of his joints and he could barely walk. Pain medication no longer rescued him. Indigestion and bloating were so prevalent and uncomfortable that he farted obsessively like an ole pack mule.

His life revolved around his taste buds. Now his life revolved around trying to feel good. His food had become poison to him. He was so miserable that he didn't want to live anymore. He was a cranky ole soul.

"Would you please slow down?", he would beg. "Just watching you is exhausting"! Me slow down? Heck I was just getting revved up.

He finally hit rock bottom. For realz. It took a lot of forethought as he forced himself to get out of bed each morning. He had a full-time job without pay just dragging his body around the house.

He shuffled his feet with each step as he attempted to create movement because pain would rip through his body like a bolt of lightning. He never knew when his heart would skip a beat or two and land him in his recliner for a few hours. He was finally ready for me to rescue him which I gladly did.

My first concern was his blood sugar. I had to get creative with meal preparations to make sure he would enjoy wholesome food as much as he did his junk food.

I knew I was safe with some of his favorites like homemade chili with beef and beans, beef vegetable soup and pot roast with vegetables. He enjoyed raw chopped onions, shredded cheese, and sour cream in his chili. I used fewer white potatoes with the pot roast because they turn to sugar quickly. Sometimes I used sweet potatoes in the crock pot with his roast. I loaded up the vegetable soup with lots of veggies and seasoned it with bay leaf, oregano, basil, and thyme. He loved the party in his mouth and would lap it up looking for more.

When he realized that he wasn't going to starve to death with healthy meals he let me incorporate small salads, a handful of potatoes instead of a plate full and one slice of buttered bread instead of two or three. Since he enjoyed sweet potatoes, he got more of those than white potatoes since they have more fiber and didn't instantly turn to sugar which in turn could spike his blood sugar.

He loved the smoothies I made with homemade yogurt, spinach, black strap molasses and a half of a banana or apple. The homemade yogurt was richer with more live probiotics than what I could buy in the store. He was enjoying low glycemic, low sugared carbohydrates, giving his body long term fuel for energy with wholesome foods while never feeling hungry. We noticed that he didn't need as much food.

The next step was getting him started on nutraceuticals, plant-based food supplements. The need for supplementation today is necessary because we can't get all the nourishment from our fruits and vegetables due to modern agricultural practices. Deleted soils, pesticides, chemical fertilizers and green harvesting deprives our food of essential nutrients.

Most supplements on the market today are synthetic and made to mimic plant-based nutrition. Our bodies are not designed to digest oyster shells, limestone, coral, sand, chalk and coal tar. They end up whole in septic tanks anyway.

His body was so glad to get the nourishment that it needed that it went right into house cleaning in the form of detoxing. This isn't always a pleasant experience. He felt worse before he felt better for about six weeks. I explained to Bill that his body was cleaning house and reminded him to drink extra water. He thought that he was allergic to healthy supplements.

He didn't understand that he was allergic to environmental and industrial waste. It was the metals, debris, pesticides and toxic prescription drugs that were being released into his bloodstream faster than his liver could handle. At least the toxins weren't coming through his skin as a rash.

We began to see little improvements in his health at first starting with healthy stools instead of chunky colored water. His body odor that previously wouldn't wash away was gone.

Acid reflux disappeared too. Yay! No more farting like a pack mule. That was so embarrassing in public because he would just let them rip as he hiked his butt cheek!

His gut was healing from all the inflammation from the production of grain alcohol that his gut was producing from the grains, sugar and Candida yeast. This meant that his food was digesting, and his body was up-taking nutrients without interference from alcohol.

He wasn't spiking his blood sugar. His food cravings disappeared, and he was full of energy. On occasion when he needed a pain pill, I gave him a massage or an Acupressure treatment.

He ditched one prescription drug after another during this transition. Doctor Jackson was so impressed that at age 75 he completely recovered his health in less than a year.

You're probably wondering how in the heck does food make this much difference. It's simple. Your cells require certain raw materials to produce energy and make healthy "babies", new cells. Every day round the clock your cells divide in order to multiply to replace themselves.

Just know that unhealthy malnourished cells divide to multiply into unhealthy cells. Nourished healthy cells divide to multiply into healthy nourished cells producing healthy tissues, organs, and skin no matter your age. Age is just a number.

This experience taught me that we can enjoy health into our golden years and has inspired me to share the good news that you don't have to suffer. You have control over your health.

Summary:

Are you sick and tired of being sick and tired of being sick and tired? Are you ready to make a lifestyle change but don't know where to start?

Since this experience with our health I've become more passionate about helping others to be more empowered to take control of their health.

I always welcome talking to people so that they can get an idea of what their life could be. If you resonate with this story and want to know if it's possible for you to go regain your health too then, I would love to communicate with you as well.

You can get some of my favorite recipes here @

https://bit.ly/RecipelessDishes

CHAPTER 2: Your Body is Hardwired to Heal Itself

"Our ills are usually our own begetting. They must be corrected by ourselves. Man is the master of his destiny, be it good or bad. Man has the inherent capacity to heal himself physically. A doctor may cleanse a wound, sew it up, bandage it well, but the natural power of the body must do the healing. Likewise, a healing process in the spirit and mind must come from within – from self-will. Others may help to cauterize the wound, suture it, and provide a clean proper environment for the healing, but the body, with the aid of the spirit, must heal itself."

Spencer W. Kimball

Did you know that 60% of Americans have a chronic disease? Did you know that 40% have 2 or more? It's also estimated that in 2030 that 83 million people will have 3 or more chronic diseases. Statistics also show that 71% of deaths worldwide are caused by poor diets making it the #1 cause of death worldwide.

Modern agricultural practices today are crafted to feed more people using less acreage. We traded quantity for quality. Mass production of food, chemical fertilizers, pesticides and green harvesting have created vitamin deficient fruits and vegetables.

Many people think of their body as a machine that will wear out with age, while unintentionally mistreating their bodies and nurturing a "we all have to die of something" type attitude. Heck some expect to break down into their 40's.

Three of my boys actually told me that they're not interested in a healthy lifestyle because in today's environment everything is unhealthy, and it doesn't matter what they do. I used to feel this way too until I learned that there are ways we can protect ourselves from the environment, pollutants and life's stressors and still be healthy. I no longer have the attitude, "I'm not going to clean my house because it's never going to stay clean anyway", with my health.

I vividly remember my first job when I was 18. I was a carhop at The Hickory House Drive Inn, in Jackson, Mississippi.

I loved this job. Cars would line up in the parking lot and I would go out and take orders and deliver their food and beverages on a tray that hung on the outside of the window of their door. They flashed their lights when they were ready for me to pick up their tray. The Hickory House was a fun hang out spot for locals.

Not only was it fun but drinks were free, and I got my food half price. I drank Coke Cola like it was water. I didn't drink water at all because it didn't have any taste. It wasn't long before my kidneys were screaming obscenities at me. I then cut way back on how much I drank.

Well, if coke cola is on the market it must not be harmful to my body, right? Wrong!

Well after years of abusing my body with fast food, soda pop and "food like substances" I was overweight, aged and unhealthy in my 40's. I thought it was normal for me to have Arthritis.

My knees would double in size with fluid, especially my right knee. I couldn't bend my knees. The joints in my fingers were stiff and painful. I had a spot in my spine that would stab me like a knife if I moved a certain way. My two big toes would throb with pain even when I wasn't walking. Little did I know that I caused this.

My grandmother had Arthritis, so I thought it was normal for me to get it too. I didn't realize that I was trashing my metabolism, disrupting my hormonal glands, feeding Candida yeast with the sugar and cheating my cells of life-giving nutrients.

I felt old and thought this was normal. By today's standards it is very normal. I was stunned that I couldn't grow strong fingernails. They got to a certain length and would break off in brittle pieces. A friend told me that soda pop would do this.

I learned that we need to keep a balance of 40% phosphorus and 60% calcium in our diet because these 2 elements work together to provide our bones, teeth, and nails with what they need to be strong and healthy.

The Phosphoric acid in soda pop is phosphorus and when we consume enough of it to be out of balance with calcium then we force phosphorus to rob the calcium out of our bones, teeth and nails creating osteoporosis and other health problems.

Even though I cut way back on soda pop I continued to eat fast food because it was a quick and easy meal. My home cooked meals came from a box most of the time because it was convenient and cheap.

It wasn't until I was 302 pounds and joined a weight loss challenge that I was ready to make my first attempt at a lifestyle change. The funny thing is that I was only doing it for the money initially. Money talks. I'm glad it does because it set me on a healing trajectory that unfolded beautifully into the career that I have today.

This is when I was introduced to nutraceuticals. I experienced their amazing effect on my body as I ditched junk food, ate whole fruits and vegetables, trimmed down, exploded my energy and felt great.

After that first competition and not winning any money, I unfortunately reverted back to my yo yo diet, while subconsciously self-sabotaging my efforts.

During the second weight loss competition I started seeing Tracy, a Naturopath, and I was mesmerized by her ability and accuracy when searching for what my body needed to heal itself.

Each visit she would begin by muscle testing as we peeled back the layers.

Muscle testing is a way to communicate energy to energy, spirit to spirit. The unspoken language of your body is energy that is easy to understand.

There are 4 muscle testing techniques that I know of to test what the body is needing. Her favorite method was having me hold a supplement and she would connect with me by touching my shoulder and she used the swaying method. She set the intention to sway forward for a yes and the intention to sway backwards for a "no". Then she would eliminate what I didn't need.

There are a few ways to muscle test to "read" the body and what it needs. I will teach my favorite methods in my online course. Muscle testing takes the guesswork out of wondering what your body needs at any given moment.

When Tracy muscle tested me, emotions would emerge, and we would do trauma releases in a fun and simple way. One time a muscle test revealed that my heart chakra was completely off to the left of my body instead of being centered in front of my heart.

Chakras are simply energy centers in our body.

I remember the day I felt it move. I was trying to forgive a nasty assault against my kids, and it was so painful that in the process of letting it go I held onto it in mid release. I could not seem to let go of the pain. It felt like a part of me was being ripped out of my chest and hanging way out in left field. It was. I couldn't breath and I felt frozen in time.

She used a green light laser in the center of my chest. I didn't know what she was doing but I trusted her skills. I vividly remember sitting on a stool with my back to the wall. After a short time, I heard this weird noise that sounded like a motor revving its engine right above my head. I cocked my head backwards to see what the ruckus was, and it was her clock. The needles were spinning counterclockwise out of control.

I looked at Tracy with that "what the heck is going on" look and we both laughed. "If I didn't see this with my own eyes, I would not believe it," I told her. She just laughed. This was the first and only time that I experienced my energy affecting an electronic device. After quite a while the motor got quiet and then the clock reset itself to the correct time. I was in shock. Energy has an electric frequency and my body's electrical frequency directly affected her clock!

As we were done with that energy correction, I explained to her why my heart was torn out of my chest. I had forgotten that I did that with my own thoughts in my effort to give my anguish to Christ. I was going through the motions but seriously couldn't let go of it as it was drifting away from me, I literally pulled back and kept the anguish. It was painful to keep but far more painful to let go of. And there it stayed until that moment.

Little did I know that I was learning energy healing and muscle testing watching Tracy as she peeled back layer after layer of traumas with me. I was inspired and wanted to learn what she knew but wasn't sure where to start.

I focused my intention on learning. Several months later a friend invited me to an essential oils class. I was awestruck with LaRee's knowledge of natural healing. She came to our little town in Idaho and taught two classes, the one on essential oils and the other one on homeopathy while advertising her energy healing classes. I recognized that this was my opportunity to learn what Tracy was doing. I jumped on it.

This is where I took a deep dive into holistic health and learned how emotions and traumas directly impact our physical and emotional health. We were taught several ways of muscle testing working with energy healing and releasing traumas using Acupressure, essential oils, homeopathy, herbs, and several other healing modalities. We learned by practicing on each other with one technique at a time with the supervision of our teacher.

As I peeled back more and more layers of emotional crap and traumas I continued to heal physically as well as emotionally. What a relief when I learned that we don't have to relive the traumas in order to release them from our nervous system and cells. I knew then that I needed to teach others what I was learning. Several of my friends want to learn so that they can help themselves and others.

I'm excited to share my signature methods of processing and releasing traumas and emotions rather than masking them with drugs, alcohol or walking back through those painful memories. There are times when we don't even need to know what trauma or emotion that is impeding progress, but our energy spirit knows.

The muscle test reveals layer by layer the energy corrections to use. This was such a relief because my own previous self-therapy was very painful as I rehashed a lot of crap the only way I knew how. I chewed on it.

We learned how to work with anxiety and depression being the emotional aspects of past traumas and fears: fear of what if..., loss..., uncertainty..., failure...and success... Low self-esteem and confidence. Self-sabotage. Feelings of unworthiness, and not being enough. Our instructor, LaRee, introduced us to Bruce Lipton.

Bruce Lipton, a stem cell biologist, then introduced us to the scientific method of how emotions create energy cysts, a code, on our DNA just like a deep wound creates a scab and then a scar on our skin. He explained that everything is energy and all energy is matter.

He showed us how all thoughts, words and emotions are finite matter that our hormones use to encode our experiences on the surface of our DNA kinda like our computers use energy frequencies to encode messages in print so that I can type these words for you to read. Since I learned that this energy piece is a missing link in so many people's healing journey, I've included this in my course material.

I'm fascinated that emotions have a chemical code that corresponds with the chemistry of an emotion. This is great news because this puts us back in control of our lives instead of outside circumstances or events. Do you remember the adage, "Control your thoughts, control your life"?

It makes sense to me that we are spirit beings having a physical experience. Our spirit is who we are. It's our thoughts, body, habits, health, intelligence, emotions and is our character. We are one with our spirit.

Some may recognize our spirit as our subconscious mind, our second brain. It's actually the other way around. Our primary brain is our energetic brain and heart where habits, desires, traumas and personality is dictating to our physical brain.

Did you know that your spirit is your automatic pilot? Just try to set goals or attempt to achieve something outside of your comfort zone and your spirit will reel you back into reality very quickly.

You may have heard the phrase, "discipline the child but don't break his spirit". Well growing up my spirit was not only broken it seemed to be destroyed. I had gotten to a point where I felt like a hollow shell of a body with no spirit. I was numb.

As my journey continued to unfold, LaRee's class then led to my attending a Cranial Sacral Therapy class where I learned to work with energy in a much different way. Cranial Sacral Therapy is a very gentle modality that works with your parasympathetic nervous system, the part of your nervous system that controls your heart, organs, breathing and calms your spirit.

After this class I decided to go to massage school where I dug deeper into Anatomy. This is where I learned to think outside the box of western medicine and inside the exciting world of natural healing using God's medicine.

I quickly learned how simple it is for our bodies to heal themselves as we listen to what they tell us. It's really quite simple working with the body's systems and hard wiring. Tia found out very quickly how simple it was to get the use of her hand back after seven years of partial paralysis.

Fresh out of massage school I didn't have the confidence to step out on my own, so I got a job as a massage therapist in a physical therapist's office. Tia came to me for a relaxing massage. When doing her intake, I questioned her for more details of what her pain points were.

She informed me that she lost the use of her right hand during a rollover car accident seven years prior as she showed me her atrophied arm from the elbow down. I could see the bones in her forearm and hand.

The jeep she was riding in rolled 6 times as she was hanging out the window. Her head brutally banged the ground six times before the jeep finally landed on her thin body pinning her to the ground.

Her doctor told her that whatever use of her hand that she got back in 2 weeks was all she could expect. She used her hand as a tray. Her thumb hadn't moved in seven years. Her index finger would bend to a 45-degree angle only. Her other three fingers took a lot of effort to slowly move down into the palm of her hand.

I explained to her that she could possibly get the use of her right hand back if we switched to Cranial Sacral Therapy. I could move the bones in her head and neck back to their proper position so that the pinched nerves that controlled her arm and hand would have freedom to fire. She opted to try.

As she laid there with her arms resting on her torso her fingers and thumbs on each hand would jump like being hit with small doses of electricity for the entire 50 minutes, more so on her paralyzed hand.

After our time was up, I asked her to show me what she could do with her hand and she quickly curled it up into a fist, moving her fingers and thumb effortlessly for the first time in 7 years. She came in for a relaxing "rub away my stress massage" and walked out with the use of her hand.

She was dumbfounded as you can imagine. She just laid there wiggling her thumb in shock. She whispered, "My thumb...my thumb...my thumb" while I was on the ceiling doing the happy dance.

She came back two more times. Upon arriving

at her third and last appointment she informed me that she gained gripping power after her second one-hour treatment. She told me that she instinctively was using her hand since she knew she could.

She unconsciously turned on the water faucet and realized it after the fact. She was shocked again. Tia then thought maybe since she could do that, then she could grip a round door knob and open the door and she did. Then she thought, "maybe I can grip an apple and peel for my daughter" and she did.

At her third appointment I used my laser on her atrophied hand and forearm to stimulate her muscles not realizing that she had no feeling from her elbow down. After the fifty-minute laser treatment she made a comment about the inside of her forearm. I put my finger on the inside of her wrist and dragged it up to her elbow and asked, "You mean right here?"? She sighed with a deep gust of air, "I can feel that!"

Can you imagine having paralysis believing your doctor that it's permanent and walking away from three one-hour treatments not only with the use of your hand but restored sensory feeling?

As a little girl, a little mother to my sisters, I

had to think for myself to figure out how to make things work. In massage school I was taught to think "outside the box" and apply my education in a way that "connects the dots" of the enormous amount of knowledge we were getting. The body will tell you what it needs. Just give it what it's asking for and it will heal itself. This is what I do, and this is what I teach in my online course.

Your body is an amazing self-healing beautiful piece of finely crafted energetic cells that are hardwired to do amazing things. Your body is anxious to heal itself but sometimes with traumas, accidents, and life in general, it gets so far off track that it needs assistance to get back to normal. It needs support.

Many have asked me to teach what I know because they aren't getting these types of results with western medicine or other therapists. Learning how to assist your body's natural healing is simple and just takes some awareness and applied principles that work and most of the time works with very few exceptions.

Summary:

We have control over our health but sometimes just don't know how to assist in healing. This is why I teach what I know.

When we know how to give our bodies what they need then our bodies will heal. This is why I'm passionate about teaching so that you can participate in your own journey.

https://bit.ly/HardwiredWorkbook

CHAPTER 3: The S.A.D. (Standard American Diet) Could Be Killing You

"Then God said, 'I give you every seed bearing plant on the face of the whole earth and every tree that has fruit and seed in it. They will be yours for food'".

Genesis 1:29

"Everything that lives and moves will be food for you. Just as I gave you the green plants, I now give you everything."

Genesis 9:3

When I was thirteen my younger sisters and I went to live with our dad and stepmother. This is when we learned domestic skills. Gardening was my favorite. We lived in the deep south, so we had a long growing season.

I fell in love with plowing the ground, making individual rows and planting seeds. I got so excited watching the seeds pop through the ground and burst magically into beautiful lush plants with juicy delicious vegetables. I loved growing my own food. Every evening we would go out to the garden and pick a basket full of food for dinner.

I remember the irresistible temptation of biting into juicy red tomatoes and letting the juice squirt all over my face and splatter all over my shirt. Our back-yard garden was rich with wholesome vegetables bursting with juicy flavor.

Before the hard frost we would be busy gathering the garden to preserve food for the winter and spring. We worked together to home can pickles from our cucumbers, beets, squashes, pumpkins, tomatoes, carrots, succotash, meatless stews that we could just add beef chunks to and so much more. We bought fruit by the boxes to bottle and freeze.

We froze our green beans, onions, dill seed, peppers, okra, a variety of beans, spinach and kale. You name it and we were growing it and putting it up to eat the rest of the year. I still love rutabagas, collard greens and turnips with turnip greens while soaking up the juices with hot cornbread dripping with butter. I can make a meal with just those. I know cornbread is made out of corn. Now that corn is mostly GMO, I don't eat this anymore. Feedlots fatten cattle with corn.

We saved seeds from our vegetables for next year's garden. We could do that because we only had heirloom seeds back then. This was before seeds were genetically modified.

Unfortunately, very few families have a backyard garden today. We have a wide variety of "food like substances" to choose from instead. Pizza, fast "food", boxed "food", snacks and energy drinks that are disruptive to our hormonal glands, digestive tracts and give us quick energy while tricking our bodies into thinking we're getting the nourishment that our cells need for optimal health.

Have you ever tasted a juicy tomato bursting with flavor straight off the vine? Do you remember the juice running down your arm and the party of flavor going off in your mouth? Now, think of the tomatoes you get in the store today that are dry and taste like cardboard. We have the same problem with fruits that are dry and grainy with a semblance of its flavors.

Society today teaches us to rely on others for our health, wellness and sustenance. We are trained to rely on others for our food. Growing your own food is easier than you think. Greenhouse gardening is making a comeback and easy to construct.

If you had a low cost way of designing and putting together a simple greenhouse using an outside wall of your house to grow your own fruits and vegetables year round, how cool would that be? There are people doing this very thing in the north. Some choose container gardening as they transition away from the Standard American Diet.

The S.A.D. comes packaged in all shapes, sizes and colors such as fast "food", frozen microwavable "meals" and boxed dead "servings" loaded with chemicals and preservatives that are devoid of vitamins, minerals and electrolytes.

Generally speaking, we are a malnourished society. Modern agricultural practices are a main contributor. Pesticides, artificial chemical fertilizers, poor soil and green harvesting which produces fruits and vegetables that lose key nutrients every year at an exponentially fast rate. We just don't get everything from our food like our grandparents did by growing their own. We simply need to supplement with quality plant-based supplements.

If all this weren't bad enough, we have the F.D.A. that is supposedly a guard dog for our health that allows harmful substances in our food such as cancer causing nitrates and other artificial preservative chemicals that disrupt our hormones and digestion.

The F.D.A. also approves red, blue, yellow and orange dyes to color food and "food like substances" to make them more appealing. These artificial dyes are made in a lab with chemicals from petroleum, a crude oil product that's also used to manufacture gasoline, diesel fuel, asphalt and tar.

Red dye is routinely made from dried bugs soaked in an alcohol as a natural ingredient in some candies, cereals, and other processed "foods" and snacks. The synthetic red dyes are known to contribute to cancer, ADHD, allergies and who knows what else.

Food manufactures resorted to a natural dye made from the Cochineal bugs that live in Peru and the Canary Islands. Local natives process the bugs for food manufacturers. Most "food like substances", aka, junk food, are dyed with this dye.

The F.D.A. also approves artificial sweeteners that are known to cause heart problems, Diabetes, and cancers. Your body doesn't know the difference between sugar and artificial sweeteners. Manufacturers are tricking you into thinking that these are a healthy alternative to sugar. It's not.

So, what's the solution?

I would recommend starting out slowly by adding whole foods into your meal plans. A side dish of lightly steamed fresh vegetables, a salad and or baked sweet potatoes, whole meats instead of processed meats and cutting back on breads, grain pastas and grains in general so that you give your cells long lasting fuel instead of temporary energy with a spike in blood sugar and extra toxins to process.

We were taught to prepare food without a recipe. To get you started experimenting with your creativity you can get my recipe-less cookbook here @ https://bit.ly/RecipelessDishes

I also invite you to become a label reader and eliminate boxed and ready made junk "foods". Phase out fast "foods' that are fattening, sugared and prepared with unhealthy fats and oils and additives. I also recommend growing your own food.

A healthy option is to shop at your local farmer's markets during the summer season. I enjoy indoor farmer's markets such as Whole Foods, Sprouts and Natural Grocers since I currently don't have a garden space of my own.

There are even memberships like Bountiful Baskets Food Co-op where you can order discounted fresh fruits and vegetables online and pick up fresh produce once a week. http://bountifulbaskets.org/

Scientists have also discovered that there are essential monosaccharides that we no longer get from our fruits and vegetables. These are missing in our S.A.D. (Standard American Diet) This will be covered in my course material because it's too much to cover in this book.

I'm healthier and more energetic today as I slide into my 70's. My motto is "age is just a number". I'm reminded to continue my 'happy aging', my journey that is filled with fun, energy and excitement. And so can you.

Happy Aging

Do you realize that the only time in your life when you want to get old is when you're young? If you're less than 10 years old you're so excited about aging that you think in fractions.

How old are you? I'm FOUR and a HALF. You're never thirty-six and a half. You're FOUR and a HALF going on FIVE.

Then you get into your teens; Now they can't hold you back, you jump to the next number. How old are you? I'm gonna be SIXTEEN. You could be twelve but you're gonna be sixteen someday.

Then the GREATEST day of your life you BECOME twenty-one. Even the words sound ceremonial... You BECOME TWENTY ONE........YESSSS!!!!!!!

Then you TURN thirty. What happened there you TURNED... Makes you sound like bad milk. Gotta throw you out?

So, you become 21; You turn 30; Then you're pushing 40, slow down; Then you reach 50; You make it to 60;

By this time, you've build up so much speed that you slide into 70;

Then you hit EIGHTY and you start slowing down.
Well, my grandmother won't even buy green bananas.
Well, it's an investment you know and maybe a bad
one. And it doesn't end there. You hit lunch; you hit
4:30. And then in your 90's you start going
backwards.

Well, I was just NINETY-TWO.

But then a strange thing happens. When you make it
to over a hundred, you become a little kid again. How
old are you? I'm a HUNDRED and a HALF... HAPPY
AGING

Summary:

The Standard American Diet could be slowly killing
you. You can get by "Fine" but wouldn't you want the
best health possible?

I'm Fine

I'm fine, I'm fine,
There is nothing the matter with me,
I'm as healthy as can be.
I have Arthritis in both of my knees,
And when I talk, I talk with a wheeze.
My pulse is weak, and my blood is thin,
But I'm awfully well for the shape I'm in.

Arch supports I have for my feet,
Or I wouldn't be able to be on the street.
Sleep is denied me, night after night,
But every morning I find I'm alright.
My memory is failing, my head's in a spin.
But I'm awfully well for the shape I'm in.

The moral is this as this tale I unfold,
That for you and me who are growing old,
It's better to say "I'm fine" with a grin,
Than to let folks know the shape we are in.

How do I know that my youth is spent?
Well my "get up and go" has done got up and went.
But I really don't mind when I think with a grin,
Of all the grand places "my get up has been."

Old age is golden, I've heard it said,
But sometimes I wonder as I get into bed.
With my ears in the drawer, my teeth in a cup,
My eyes on the table until I wake up.

Ere sleep comes over me. I say to myself,
Is there anything else I could lay on the shelf?

Author Unknown

CHAPTER 4: Emotions Alter Your DNA Expression... Epigenetics

"The scientific knowledge derived from genetics, epigenetics and neuroscience, should be used to enhance the power of meditation and to eliminate the sufferings of humanity."

Amit Ray

Do you remember basic science when you were in elementary school and your teacher taught you the basic structure of life is atoms, electrons, neutrons, and protons? Do you remember learning that an atom is the smallest unit of life?

Did you know that when scientists examined the composition of an atom there was no physical material? Yup! That's right. When examined under a microscope the atom is spinning energy. The organelles inside the nucleus of the cell are also spinning energy and not physical tangible particles.

Your body is a busy community of 50 Trillion

compressed cells of spinning energy each with its own brain and operating system of organelles and miniature organs, suspended in a jelly-like cytoplasm of spinning energy. These organelles are miniature versions of the tissues and organs of your own body.

They have their own functional equivalent to your body's functioning systems. Each microscopic cell has its own digestive, nervous, respiratory, excretory (waste disposal), muscular, endocrine (hormonal), reproductive, skeletal, circulatory, and immune, and its own integumentary system (skin).

Just as we respond to our environment and create a memory, each of our cells likewise responds to its environment and creates a memory while responding to their environment via our nervous and hormonal systems.

Your individual cells mimic your physical - energetic body as you are the sum of all of your trillions of cells and energy. What impacts your cells impacts you and your health on the cellular level.

Each of your cells are an intelligent being that can live, divide to multiply, and thrive outside of your body in a petri dish with a chemical version of blood.

Bruce Lipton, a stem cell biologist, experimented with the environment of a single stem cell in a petri dish. After this stem cell divided to multiply into 50,000 identical stem cells he took 3 petri dishes and mixed three different mediums to mimic 3 different chemical mediums for each petri dish. To his astonishment each petri dish made 3 different trays of tissues. This groundbreaking experiment was at the beginning of the new field of Epigenetics.

You control the chemical composition of your blood with your emotional reactions to your environment. This in turn determines which hormones you create that are released into your blood.

This new science proves that the environment of your cells directly impacts the characteristics of your cells and that you can change those characteristics by changing the chemistry of your blood.

You alter the chemistry of your blood with nutrition, toxins, vaccines, traumas, injuries, thoughts, words, beliefs, attitudes, laughter, sunlight and lack of sunlight which are all simply your emotional and physical responses to your environment.

Everything is made of energy. Everything. Energy can never be destroyed but it can be altered. For instance, 2 molecules of hydrogen and 1 molecule of oxygen energy makes water. You can't destroy water, but you can alter it into steam, ice, hail, fog and snow just by changing its environment.

The same principle applies to your body. Thoughts, beliefs and emotions are energy. Your nervous system is energy and relies on the energy field of your hormones to alter your blood chemistry that alters your cells just like in Bruce Lipton's experiment.

Let's say for an example that you suffer from depression and or anxiety. The energy of your thoughts changes the chemical composition of your blood. A code is generated that imprints on the surface of your DNA like a scar from a physical wound on the surface of your skin.

These emotional scars or energy cysts are the memories stored on the surface of your DNA until you release them. You do this with the reverse of how you created them to begin with - thoughts, emotions, words, meditation, music, etc.

Summary:

We are not victims of our circumstances, environment or traumas. Life is full of lessons and opportunities disguised as problems. When we flip our mindset and use these opportunities as growth opportunities instead of a chance to curl up and sulk then we can alter our gene expressions - our programming. Our emotional reactions become proactive instead of reactive.

"Be grateful for all the crap you have to take in life because it's the fertilizer that makes you grow!"

Dexter Yager

You can get my workbook companion to this book @:

https://bit.ly/HardwiredWorkbook

CHAPTER 5: Rewriting Your DNA Expressions

"What would your life be like if you learned that you are more powerful than you've ever been taught?"

Bruce Lipton, stem cell biologist

"In all the universe there can be no such things as luck or fate; every action, every thought is governed by law. Behind every bit of good fortune the causes that we ourselves have sometime, somewhere set in motion. Behind all ill fortune we will find the energy, we ourselves, have generated. Every cause must have a certain definite effect, there is no dodging the results, we reap what we sow with exact mathematical precision"

Venice Bloodworth, PhD Psychologist

My grandmother Sara told me that I was the easiest little girl in the world to cry. I cried over every little thing. I had such low self-esteem that the first word out of my mouth was, "I can't". She tried for a few years to convince me that there was no such word as "can't". I didn't trust myself or anyone else. I felt powerless against the monster I called "life".

My little girl felt worthless and incapable of achieving anything. Life was overwhelming and not worth living. The weight of the world was heavy as I felt forced to survive. My only ray of hope was my grandmother. I knew she loved me, but I didn't get to spend much time with her.

"Go get the dictionary off the shelf, Vicki" she finally said one day. "Now look up the word "can't". "This would be easy," I thought to myself. I learned how to alphabetize words in the third grade. "I'll show her," I thought as I rushed over to get the dictionary. Well, guess what? I couldn't find it. Back in the 1950's there were no contractions in the dictionary. She tricked me.

"I can only find 'can'", I informed her as I plundered through the dictionary. "See, since there's no such word as 'can't', then you CAN. You can do anything you put your mind to. You just need to put in the effort, and you will figure it out," she would insist. This little seed of 'can' became my life's motto. Just let someone tell me that I can't accomplish something and I'll make sure they watch me doing it!

My grandmother sits on my shoulder even today, sixty years later, nudging me on. When I sat in class learning energy healing, I had no idea what I had gotten myself into. Tracy made it seem so easy and effortless.

I was determined to understand how to continue to heal from traumas naturally and without drugs or psychotherapy. I was so tired of reliving all of that crappy pain every time I got triggered by a life's event. I was tired of living with the debilitating traumas that triggered me into depression, anxiety and lethargy. I was tired of being suicidal. I was tired of dragging my body through life. I was just tired.

I watched others living a successful happy life and I wanted this for myself and my family. As I studied and peeled back the layers of traumas, I discovered that I was my own worst enemy. I struggled to overcome the demons inside my head that convinced me that I was not enough and that I had no value. I had two husbands who reminded me that I wasn't worth much and was nothing without them. The sad thing is that I believed them. My own beliefs held me captive.

So here I was sitting in class fumbling around in an arena that seemed very unconventional. I felt lost because I had no foundational knowledge of how the body heals itself and I was confused. I didn't want to make mistakes. I had to make the information my own in order to understand what I was learning.

The more I learned the more I realized that I was learning how to use God's medicine. This is when I was first introduced to Bruce Lipton. He explained to us how emotions are energetic matter, finite energy molecules that can alter our DNA expressions.

He explained how we are "skin covered petri dishes". This means we literally alter our blood, cells and body with food, emotions, thoughts, words, and our environment which then imprints the surface of our DNA with a code.

Our DNA expression influences our mood, character, thoughts, beliefs and is who we are. Once I truly grasped the understanding of how this all works, I began using my power to rewrite my gene expression and assisting others with my signature treatments. I began responding to life and its many opportunities in a more positive and productive way instead of reacting with self-destructive patterns.

It was much easier for me to react in self punishing actions. You may have heard the phrase, "discipline the child but don't break his spirit". Well growing up my spirit was not only broken it seemed to be destroyed. I had gotten to a point where I felt like a hollow shell of a body with no spirit. I was numb with no feelings and had actually put up a shield to protect me from further attacks.

It was during a muscle testing exercise in my energy healing class twenty-six years later that one of my fellow students discovered my energetic shield. She said it was made out of metal. I had to laugh because I forgot that I put it there. I emotionally put it in place back in the 1980's and yes, it was made out of metal like you see in the Gladiator movies.

When something like an insult would come at me, I would visualize it bouncing off of the shield and back to the person who slung it at me. I immediately took it down and opened my heart to others as I peeled off another layer of emotional trauma.

Everything is energy. Emotions are energy.

Energy is a finite matter. Your emotional reactions to life create chemical codes using your hormones and nervous system to create energy cysts as a "boo boo" just like your skin forms a scar after an injury. The deeper the injury the deeper the scar.

The deeper the trauma, the deeper the energy cysts. The energy of emotions attaches to the surface of your DNA like code on a website and stays there until you release and clear it out. You clear them out with thoughts, words, emotions, and intentions. You will learn techniques using Acupressure, breathwork and meditation in my online class.

You can be your own worst enemy or your own best friend depending on how you respond to life and its many opportunities that are disguised as problems, injuries, and traumas. You and you alone control your destiny with your emotions, thoughts, and actions. This is quantum physics simplified.

As I explore more into quantum physics the true meaning of "everything is energy" opens up a whole new world of awareness and perceptions. I'm learning the true meaning of how the energy of emotions carves out individual unique paths to health.

This explains why there are so many variables in similar environments. Your emotional reactions are based on a combination of your ancestral genetics, epigenetics (stored ancestral emotions), environment, self-image and what you tell yourself throughout the day.

We are energy beings having a physical experience. Even our physical bodies are made of compressed energy. Bruce Lipton explains this so well in his short YouTube video.

https://www.youtube.com/watch?v=zodg4WwBovc

Since you are ultimately in control of your own energy through your thoughts, emotional reactions, perceptions, words, and actions then you control your own fate. You are not at the mercy of a disease, illness, or financial demise. You are not at the mercy of the economy. You are only at the mercy of yourself.

"If ye have the faith as a grain of a mustard seed, ye shall say unto this mountain, remove hence to yonder place; and it shall be removed; and nothing shall be impossible unto you." Mathew 17:20

What mountain is standing in your way that you want to remove? What opportunity is waiting for you on the other side of that mountain?

Remember back when you were a child and, in your imagination, you would create imaginary friends? You would dream of what you would be when you grew up. You fantasized what it would be like to be an adult and fly all over the world as a very important executive. Would you pretend that you were a doctor, scientist or famous inventor?

What is your childhood dream that is just waiting for you to pursue? Or has that changed? What's stopping you from pursuing your dreams? What would you do if you knew you couldn't fail?

It's really up to you.

This concept also gives a deeper meaning to the quote:

"Watch your thoughts for they become your words; watch your words for they become your actions: watch your actions for they become your habits; watch your habits for they become your character; watch your character for it becomes your destiny."

When I vowed as a little 8-year-old girl that I

would grow up and save children from childhood abuse I had no idea I would be the first one that I saved. My personal journey from victim to holistic therapist has been truly transformational as I grasped the understanding of how to use my own power to heal my little girl and assist others in doing the same.

Using your own power to heal is far more powerful and longer lasting and transformative than any other method. This is why I work "with" my clients and not let them rely solely on me to "fix" them.

Did you know that your emotional reactions to life's events are the most powerful events that impact your health? Unknowingly you create your own demise with your emotions. These can be a stressor or a healer. Emotions trigger a hormonal response that alters your blood chemistry which in turn alters your DNA expressions that is a "compass" for your health.

Cortisol is your flight for life hormone that shuts down digestion, hunger, thinking, sleep, metabolism and sex drive. It also releases glucose into your bloodstream to provide you energy, triggering an insulin response which can lead to weight gain or unhealthy weight loss.

Stress can lead to most diseases such as Heart disease, Autoimmune disorders, anxiety, depression, high blood pressure, Type 2 Diabetes, Cushing Syndrome and can cause inflammation while compromising your immune system.

The 5 most stressful events in your life are:
1) death of a loved one
2) divorce
3) moving
4) major illness
5) job loss

January 4th, 2018, I walked away from my second unhealthy marriage with $400 and what I could put in my little car. I was at a breaking point emotionally and mentally while feeling there were no other options.

I had no idea of where I was going to live or what I was going to do. I walked away from a property that I truly loved. I had just invested 2 ½ years of savings, another 2 ½ years of sweat equity, and along with possessions that I dreamed of having for years, all for my sanity.

I vividly remember wishing I would just stop

breathing and "go home" in my sleep. The jaws of depression had swallowed my head and had its teeth clamped deep into my neck and shook me to the very core of my being. I would sit for hours musing myself unmotivated to get up and do anything. This went on for a solid six months. I was angry that I had put myself in this predicament.

I didn't feel like I had a purpose for being here and wondered why God didn't just take me home. I spent a lot of time in my head feeling like I was drifting aimlessly into the blackness of space.

Breathing was a difficult task and seemed like too much work. Often, I couldn't talk without crying. There seemed to be no end in sight. I moved six times that first year. Fortunately, I ended up staying with loving supportive friends who nurtured me the best they knew how. They really didn't know what to do with me or how to help me. Time dragged on.

I slowly began changing my emotional reactions to my circumstances, mood and attitude with music.

Every day I listened to motivational songs of hope. I especially loved listening to children sing. I sang church hymns. I would soak up music with my eyes closed and with my intention, I would bathe my cells in the words and melodies of each carefully selected song. I could feel the healing with the various energy frequencies.

At that time, I didn't realize that I was altering my blood chemistry and ultimately my epigenetic expressions. I was lapping up huge helpings of delicious Dopamine, my feel-good hormone. Music was food for my soul as I gorged on Dopamine.

Audrey Draper, music intern describes this much better than I can:

"There is something profoundly magic about the power of music. Music is a universal language. It allows us to communicate with ANYONE without the requirement of spoken language.

It is connecting and uniting across cultures and language barriers. It also allows us to connect to ourselves; our heart - our lifeblood. One reason we feel such a deep connection to music is because of rhythm.

We have an internal rhythm that keeps us alive everyday - our heartbeat. When we listen to and engage with music that resonates with us, we are connecting with the deepest, most primal part of our humanity.

Music touches the heart and the soul in ways words will never be able to describe, much like our pain can affect us in the most deep and often dark ways that we cannot fully express with words.

When we feel something so heavy and indescribable, we often turn to the expressive arts as they too make us feel things we cannot express verbally. Music can and should be used as a powerful healing tool." Audrey Draper, MTI (Music Therapy Intern)

During this time, I subscribed to Kyle Cease and his motivational transformational standup comedy. I immersed myself in his guided meditations and flooded my whole being with all the inspirational messages that I needed.

His humor mixed with inspiration and logic gave me food for thought. I learned how to calm my soul to hold space for my emotions while not passing judgement or finding fault. I looked for the opportunities in my demise while letting those emotions work their way out.

This quiet time with myself was calming to my nerves while I changed my self-destructive thoughts into healthy nurturing thoughts of love, healing and forgiveness. He and his community of others who were hurting became my family as I could relate to their stories of triumph over traumas.

Then one day the dark cloud lifted off of me and I found myself back on Earth counting my blessings. It felt like a very physical experience. This was a major milestone for me. You see, I've started over more times than I care to count, losing material possessions that I had worked so hard to get. And here I was again getting to start all over at the ripe young age of 66 with no savings, no home of my own, possessions that I can fit into my car and lots of uncertainty.

I put my faith in God that He would work things out to help me put me back together while I learned my lessons.

So here I am with a new lease on life when I met Andrea Scarborough on Facebook. I met her just as I was coming out of HELL but wasn't put back together emotionally or mentally. She offered me her Empower Hour and it was just what I needed. Andrea knew just how to help me get back up and running again with self-esteem, confidence, energy and zest for life. We became instant friends. She came into my life just at the right time.

After years of working with those with mental illness she has developed her signature method of asking the right questions to get to the right answers. She introduced me to me in a way that I had never experienced before. I saw me through my mess. She saw my unique awesomeness. She will see your unique awesomeness as well and I highly recommend her to you. Here's a link for those who don't have the ebook: http://bit.ly/PSS-Empower-Hour.

Well, with that magic carpet ride, I put my big girl panties back on and took my life back. I didn't realize it at the time, but she empowered me to use my own power to heal myself AGAIN.

I applied the principles that I teach. I was recoding my DNA expressions with gratitude for what I had while releasing anger, regrets and sadness. I focused on the benefits of the lessons learned. Wisdom, compassion, patience and starting over wiser and stronger revealed itself.

I turned my attention to assisting my clients in getting well while setting new goals and my bright future. It felt like the weight of the world was off my shoulders. I felt 40 pounds lighter as I embraced my new adventures.

I got to start over with 40 years of experience

in getting back up after getting knocked down time after time after time and the valuable wisdom from those experiences. I started over with strength, compassion, empathy for others, patience, grit, and a "can do" positive winning attitude. What I thought was a mess was truly a blessing in disguise.

I soon realized that I was much stronger and happier than I had been in years. All it took was a mind shift and redirecting my thoughts, feelings, words, and emotions as I let go of regrets and focused on my next adventure. This didn't need to take a year, but I hear that's the average time after divorce or major loss.

Now I have skills and tools to make my turnaround instant as I hop from one steppingstone to another, letting life unfold while making the best out of each experience.

"You never know how strong you are until being strong is the only choice you have."

Fast forward and here I've had an amazing 2019 with earning an incentive trip to Costa Rica by assisting others in regaining their health. I'm heading into 2020 writing this book and launching my online course teaching others my signature method of what I've learned with natural healing. It feels like an amazing year already.

Then... the Coronavirus disrupted life as we know it. I'm getting creative in learning to use the virtual world to reach out and help heal my human family. When life gets disruptive it gives us opportunities to expand our creativeness.

I'm learning to take my business online where I can reach more people who are searching for answers and resources. I get to expand my outreach in ways not possible offline. How are you using this opportunity? What's your next move?

Summary:

The Dash
by Linda Ellis

"I read of a man who stood to speak at the funeral of a friend. He referred to the dates on the tombstone from the beginning... to the end.

He noted that first came the date of birth and spoke of the following date with tears, but he said that what mattered most of all was the dash between those years.

For that dash represents all that time that they spent alive on earth and now only those who loved them know what that little line is worth.

For it matters not how much we own, the cars...the house...the cash. What matters most is how we live and love and how we spend our dash.

So, think about this long and hard; Are there things you'd like to change? For you never know how much time is left that can still be rearranged.

To be less quick to anger and show appreciation more and love the people in our lives like we've never loved before.

If we treat each other with respect and more often

wear a smile...remembering that this special dash might only last a little while.

So, when your eulogy is being read, with your life's actions to rehash, would you be proud of the things they say about how you lived your dash?"

It's how you overcome great tragedies that causes you to switch gears and jump track from fate to destiny.

"If you spend your entire life with the mentality that my traumas have screwed me up and this is why I am the way I am instead of learning how to heal and grow from your traumas, then you are your own problem."

Gaia

Learning to respond to life's twists and turns in a proactive healthy way gives you the opportunities to use your experiences to strengthen and empower you forward into your greatness.

You can get a complimentary copy of my workbook
companion to this book here @
https://bit.ly/HardwiredWorkbook

CHAPTER 6: APPLIED ANATOMY 101- Understanding Your Body

"If my body was a car, I would be trading it in for a newer model. I've got bumps, dents, scratches & my headlights are out of focus. My gearbox is seizing up & it takes me hours to reach maximum speed. I overheat for no reason and everytime I sneeze, cough or laugh either my radiator leaks or my exhaust backfires!"

My first introduction to Anatomy was a fun childhood song, "Dry Bones (Dem Bones)". Do you remember this song?

https://www.youtube.com/watch?v=cLi55MV04a8

Dem bones, dems bone dem dry bones,

Dem bones, dem bones dem dry bones,

Dem bones, dem bones dem dry bones,

Now shake dem skeleton bones!

The toe bone's connected to the foot bone,

The foot bone's connected to the ankle bone,

The ankle bone's connected to the leg bone,

Now shake dem skeleton bones!

The leg bone's connected to the knee bone,
The knee bone's connected to the thigh bone,
The thigh bone's connected to the hip bone,
Now shake those skeleton bones!

Dem bones, dems bone dem dry bones,
Dem bones, dem bones dem dry bones,
Dem bones, dem bones dem dry bones,
Now shake dem skeleton bones!

The hip bone's connected to the back bone,
The back bone's connected to the neck bone,
The neck bone's connected to the head bone,
Now shake those skeleton bones!

The finger bone's connected to the hand bone,
The hand bone's connected to the arm bone,
The arm bone's connected to the shoulder bone,
Now shake dem skeleton bones!

Dem bones, dems bone dem dry bones,
Dem bones, dem bones dem dry bones,
Dem bones, dem bones dem dry bones,
Now shake dem skeleton bones!

Well as you can imagine this introduction to Anatomy was not good enough for massage. We took a much deeper dive.

The first thing our Anatomy teacher asked all of us was, "What's your biggest dread in learning Anatomy"? I raised my hand and replied, "Learning Latin." He shook his head yes. He informed us that all of the parts of the body were named by the early Latin Anatomists and yes, we would be learning some Latin.

We learned the Latin name for each muscle, the "bony landmarks" that the tendons of each muscle attached to, the function of each of those muscles, the name of the function and the exact location of each muscle in 4 semesters. You can imagine how intense that was, especially for this 61-year-old who hadn't been to college in over 20 years.

This was like being in Kindergarten learning our ABC's one muscle group at a time. I didn't appreciate learning all of that just to give a massage. Little did I realize at the time that I was being prepped for transformational healing for my clients. I was learning how to get to the source of a physical imbalance, trauma and injury while working towards recovery, not just rubbing down bodies.

I remember being fresh out of massage school and meeting Mary. She came to the door bent in half and twisted off to her right side. She was my first transformational success.

As Mary slowly struggled her way onto my massage table and finally came to rest on my table exhausted by the struggle. She was curled up in a little ball unable to lie flat. She informed me that when she went to bed at night, she would prop herself up with numerous pillows to support her twisted and mis-shaped body.

My first goal before we could get much work done was to straighten out her body. Structural class was fresh on my mind as I whittled away the tensions in her little body moving from spot to spot just like a wood carver whittles away what he doesn't want in order to produce a masterpiece.

After about an hour, I stepped back to reassess what should be next. And then it hit me. "Mary, do you realize that you are lying flat on my table," I asked her with a big smile. "Yes, I do", she said with the first smile since we started. "How exciting is this?

How do you feel?" I asked. She grinned from ear to ear, "I feel good!".

Then there was Russell.

When I first met Russ, he was shuffling in an attempt to walk bent over holding onto his walker. His doctor couldn't find anything wrong with him. He was so miserable with chronic pain. He tossed and turned all night trying to get comfortable but couldn't sleep. No position lasted very long before pain would shoot through his low back and down into his legs. He couldn't stand up straight.

He had trouble sitting from a stooped position and stooping from a sitting position. He could barely reach his feet to put his shoes and socks on. Pain would shoot into his buttocks and down his legs. He swore that he had sciatica. He was miserable all the time.

He trusted me to a point but after 2 sessions of Psoas work, he was convinced that his pelvic bone was splitting apart and going to fall off of his spine and legs.

"I'm just going to cancel my next appointment and go see a specialist to see if there's something he can do for me," he informed me. "I'm going to see if there's a test they can do to see if my bones are separating and splitting apart," he continued.

"It's your Psoas muscle," I relentlessly assured. Finally, he gave in and kept his appointment with me. Each session was more and more tolerable as his walking muscle was loosening its grip on his spine.

It wasn't long before he ditched his walker and was sleeping peacefully at night. He would greet me at the door with a big smile on his face thanking me for my persistence and patience.

Many people ask me what sets me apart from other therapists. I learned how to connect the dots of everything I learned with all of my education. I think outside the box to tailor a treatment to each client's needs. I focus on targeting the problem area beginning with the most painful first working around the body.

I learned how to move bones to free up pinched nerves that control movement, tingling, and numbness. I use Cranial Sacral Therapy to regulate and eliminate pain, headaches, sinus pressure, TMJ pain, and other imbalances. Connecting dots with

Anatomy allows us to figure out how to assist the body to heal itself. I include these techniques in my online course.

This is how I helped Tia regain the use of her partially paralyzed hand. As the jeep she was riding in caught the edge of the shoulder the jeep began rolling down the embankment. The chest strap was broken, and she hung out the window and brutally banged her head each time the jeep struck the ground, compressing the nerves in her head. It was a miracle that she lived.

Contrary to popular belief, you do not have a "hard head". You have numerous bones in your head separated by cartilage that are easily moved and misplaced by even the slightest bump. Any one or more of your 12 cranial nerves can get compressed, pinching off your ability to send a signal to your body. This can be a cause of seizures, numbness, tingling, restless legs, cold hands and feet and muscle spasms or any combination of the above depending on the degree of the impingement.

In Tia's case, she had numbness from her elbow down and partial paralysis in her right hand with no gripping power. After listening to her account of the accident I informed her that she pinched nerves in her head that went down into her arm.

I explained to her that my education taught me that nerves control muscle and muscle controls movement and that it's possible that she could get the use of her hand back. Her doctor told her that whatever movement and feeling she got back in 2 weeks was all she could expect. However, this did not make sense to me with my study of Anatomy.

So here she is 7 years later coming to me for a relaxing massage and walking out an hour later with the use of her hand. Can you imagine the shock she must have been in?

After her second one-hour session she regained gripping power and in her last 1 one hour session she got the feeling back in her arm and hand with the therapeutic healing of a red light laser to stimulate her previously pinched nerves.

Then there is Joby's friend who wants to remain anonymous. He was in several fights as a reporter for non-mainstream news. He got his face rearranged a few times and his nose was misplaced off to the right of his face.

His Psoas muscle, his walking muscle that stores traumas and emotions, was locked up too. After opening up his Psoas muscle and freeing up his back pain while giving his digestive organs space to function properly, he felt great. He carried around a cold box container to keep some special pain meds so that he could make it through each day. After his treatment he told me that he didn't think he would need those anymore as he could breath and felt "opened up" in his abdomen. He was free from pain.

At the end of that treatment when working on his neck I looked down at his face and noticed that his nose was off centered and I informed him that I could straighten his nose but it would take about an hour.

At first, he was excited at the possibility. When he returned the next day, he was pessimistic. He even told me that he didn't think I could do it but was willing to try. After an hour of moving bones in his head and palate, I informed him that his nose was centered on his face again.

Oh my gosh you should have seen him. He went into the bathroom to check out his nose. He was in there so long that I thought he "fell in". He came out dancing and hootin' and a hollerin'. "My nose, my nose! Look what she did for my nose"! He thought it was a miracle but it's simple.

You see, you have several bones that your nose is attached to. When these bones are misplaced your nose follows the direction of the misplacement. Put the bones back in their proper position and your nose moves with them. It seems like magic but it's really working with Anatomy.

Little 3 ½ year old Jonathan fell hard a few times off of the rocking chair and hit his head on the hard floor and almost passed out last fall. He lost bladder control and was wetting his pants because he didn't know when he needed to go to the bathroom until it was too late. His mother wanted me to check him out and see if I could help him.

They are Amish and prefer alternative treatments to Western medicine, so she didn't take him to the doctor. She asked me to figure out what was wrong. I instantly knew that he pinched nerves in his head. It only took one Cranial Sacral Therapy treatment freeing up the bones in his head and neck to correct the imbalance. Over a period of 2 weeks he was going to the bathroom on his own again and not wetting his bed.

He also splayed his left leg out to get comfortable on my table. This told me that he threw his hip out. A little gentle tractioning on his pelvis and leg put his leg back in its socket. You should have seen the big smile on his face as he couldn't take his eyes off of me. He felt good.

Have you ever stubbed your toe and it hurt so bad that it hurt to walk even barefoot? Forget about putting a shoe on. You are pinching a nerve as well as your tissues tightening up to force you to put your foot up and stay off of it. Well Tom dropped something very heavy on his toe through his shoe and the pain was a constant miserable throb.

He declined my help because touching his toe was extremely painful. Well, his wife had a different plan. She insisted that I help him. We both walked up on him, her behind him and me in front.

He squirmed wondering what we were up to. She grabbed his arms as I grabbed his leg. "What are you doing?" he demanded. "She's going to help your toe", his wife insisted. "I promise I won't hurt you". He gave in.

I simply put one finger lightly on the top of his purple toe and another one on the bottom and asked him, "Does this hurt"? "No, it doesn't", he said as he completely relaxed. "I'm just going to do some tractioning until I feel the adjustment", I explained to him. I did a very light gentle constant tractioning towards me until I felt his joint readjust itself. It felt like a little tremor, a little vibration. He felt nothing as we talked the whole time.

I had him stand up and take a few steps. He looked back at me with that "hmmm" look on his face and said, "It doesn't hurt". He continued to walk all the way around to the other side of the pool table and said to his wife Cora, "It doesn't hurt. What did she do? What did she do?" as he slung his glasses across the pool table. He turned and looked at me and asked, "What did you do? It doesn't hurt!".

I had the pleasure of assisting Vickie Gould with a 2-hour treatment at a recent retreat we both attended. She had been anxiously awaiting her turn to get a treatment. Her neck and Psoas muscles were locked up and it was creating chronic discomfort and pinched nerves. I spent an hour on her upper body and an hour on her lower body. Here's her version of her treatment that she posted on Facebook:

"Vicki, I was thinking about you this morning as I went to my weekly 2-hour massage. I think you might've put my chiropractor out of business (well at least for me) because that ONE session of bodywork you did has lasted a LONG TIME! You really are "magic hands"!

I don't know if you know this, but even though my insurance covers my massages and I've been going since around 2010 EVERY WEEK since all my Chronic Lyme Disease issues, I have to fulfill my $5000 deductible every year with my chiro/massage visits before insurance kicks in to cover it all.

I think you just saved me $5000! No, I KNOW you saved me $5000. Even though you're in CO, it would be sooooo worth it for me to even fly to you to be worked on. I feel like you could be the secret to the Hollywood stars!"

When you understand Anatomy and work with the natural functions of the body then the body responds and heals itself.

Then there's my client who prefers I not use her name. She approached me to see if I could help her. She was looking for relief from physical imbalances that were several years old and not going away. I'll let her tell you her story:

"For years my back, neck and shoulders had caused me problems. Minor, but still significant enough to hinder and alter certain activities I enjoyed or wished to participate in. I'm sure poor posture, bad habits, pregnancy and nursing, packing around babies and small children all contributed to this and compounded my problems.

I hadn't been flexible enough to touch my toes in over 6 years. My shoulders were starting to round more, and I looked like an old lady–unable to straighten my shoulders and back like I used to. I had severe back and hip issues at the start and throughout my 3rd pregnancy.

At one point I couldn't move or walk and required help around the home and walking sticks to move around during the day. I couldn't lift my baby in and out of the crib. I slept on the floor for 2 ½ weeks, lying flat on my back even though I'm a side sleeper, because the pain was so awful. Note, all of the bedrooms were upstairs and I had to sleep in the living room for those couple of weeks.

My almost 4-year-old had to help dress me. Using the bathroom was excruciating to get down or especially back up from a sitting position. I required help or the use of the hiking poles-all the whole while I screamed in agony. This pain would subside, and I would forget about it since it wasn't screaming at me. Every once in a while, it let me know it was still there. I would baby it, be careful, "get better" and move on. This was the same pattern for several years.

After several months of treatment with Vicki, I began to see notable changes. My flexibility was greatly improved! It felt so amazing to finally bend over and touch my toes again! I attribute this to her knowledge of the body and also being in tune with mine.

Doing stretches has been a vital part of this process. The times I go without stretching, or skimping on them, my body starts to tighten and sometimes even seize up again. We're still making progress and working on my "issues". I'm excited to get mobility and flexibility back like I once had and not hobble around like an old woman."

These are all examples of why I'm teaching a simple version of Anatomy in my course material so that you will understand how your body works so that you can participate in your own natural healing.

Summary:

Your body is hardwired to heal itself. Sometimes your body gets so far off track that it needs a little assistance. Applied knowledge is power.

Understanding how your body works, working with nature the way your body understands will get you expedited healing. Sometimes it's just a matter of knowing what to do to help your body. This is why I'm excited to share my knowledge and expertise.

You get some Applied Anatomy in my free workbook companion here @ https://bit.ly/HardwiredWorkbook

CHAPTER 7: EMF Radiation, a Toxic Poison
by Samantha Villipu

Introduction to EMFs:

Humans evolved on Earth over millions of years ago, with our cells tuned to the natural electromagnetic frequencies of the Sun and Earth; there is an entire symphony of biological processes that need to occur, all at specific times, commanded by the changing light and magnetic field around us.

If the timing of these processes is distorted, our body won't have optimal repair, leading to symptoms like insomnia, anxiety, headaches, fatigue, brain-fog, etc. and eventually an outright diagnosis of a disease, such as Diabetes, Parkinson's, Cancer, and so on.

Since electricity was first brought into the cities in 1910, we've been living in artificial light and EMG (electromagnetic) environments which interfere with our cells' ability to detect the natural frequencies that they require. We do have a built-in resilience, but multigenerational epigenetic damage and ever-increasing exposure (5G anyone?) has brought us to a tilting-point and we are seeing this manifest in nearly everyone around us being sick.

Quantum BioPhysics is a new branch of science that isn't taught in medical school, so very few doctors are aware of this, in fact, you now know more about how the body functions than 99% of doctors!

Electricity and wireless technology isn't going away soon, so it's our job to learn how to use it wisely - making choices that give our cells the signals they require for natural regeneration processes to be restored." ~ Samantha Vilppu, Shamanic Living LLC (for more info, visit www.SamanthaVilppu.com/EMF)

How I came to this point of teaching about EMFs:

1996 - It was my final year in college. I was graduating at the top of my class in Architectural Engineering (Solar emphasis), with a 4.2 GPA. I had been walking 3 times a day and was in fitness, essentially at the top of my game.

Then something changed. One day I went out for my mid-day walk and about a block away, I became weak to the point that I couldn't even walk home. I crawled back to my apartment. I had to sleep at least 14 hours a day and while awake, I couldn't do more than 3 "things" in a day such as get the mail, cook lunch, etc.

Lots of lab work and several doctors later, there was no clear diagnosis for what I was experiencing. They decided to label it "Mono" and move on. It lasted several months and then I seemed to have a partial recovery as I graduated and moved out of state. Unfortunately, the symptoms never completely disappeared. Symptoms would come and go somewhat unpredictably.

Eventually, I was labeled with chronic fatigue, depression, fibromyalgia, hypothyroidism, and a few other things. Needless to say, my functioning was far lower than I had been experiencing during my college years. I spent the next 23 years in this interim testing out several modalities and treatments in hopes that they would help me feel better. Of course, some worked better than others and provided a sense of relief, but nothing that was restoring me back to who I know myself to be.

Then one day in 2019, in a Facebook group for a course that taught several actions that helped one person, I noticed that this person was encouraging the use of "wearable" devices that track sleep or brain wave patterns. While I am all for being able to track these states, these devices are usually Bluetooth and I already was aware that I would get a headache whenever Bluetooth was turned on near me.

I asked if he knew of any that weren't Bluetooth based. A fellow member commented with a snarky remark that Bluetooth was NO different than WiFi and that if I could handle WiFi then I should be able to handle Bluetooth.

With my architectural engineering training, I was aware of electromagnetic radiation but hadn't given it much attention during this time. I was even in circles with the top EMF engineers back around 2000. For some reason, I couldn't bring myself to invest the $350 to purchase an EMF meter that would measure even one of the several fields I needed to know about in my environment.

This Facebook remark triggered me into refreshing my prior engineering understanding of EMFs as well as gaining clarity around the swirling list of EMF meters on the market. They all stated what they measured but from the standpoint of an 'outsider' it was impossible to know if they would measure what I needed them to. So, I took a day and delved into gaining more clarity around all of the frequencies and ranges that these meters coveted. What I found was that NONE of the 50 or so meters listed on one of the popular EMF supply sites actually looked satisfactory.

Fortunately, a quick online search turned up a review for a brand of meter that this company wasn't offering, describing it as "The best meter for 2019". Long story short, it really did cover all of the fields and ranges that I was looking for, all for $125... so, I finally allowed myself to buy the EMF meter (after wanting one for 20 years)!

When I received it and began using it, I noticed the most interesting thing – when my symptoms were higher, the meter was reading higher; when my symptoms were lower, the meter was reading lower.

So, I took some actions to deliberately create a space where the electromagnetic fields were lower, and wow – I began to feel better than I had in years!

At the same time as I was having this "reawakening", I was hearing things about the new 5G cell-phone systems that were about to roll out, so I began to dive in to research it a bit to gain clarity around what we would be dealing with.

What turned up in my research wasn't only about 5G, but instead about how our cells are affected by all forms of EMF radiation. It seemed a little "out there" to me at first, but because of the neurosurgeon status of the person teaching this information, I opted to listen more to evaluate it at a deeper level. What I was discovering was "the other side of the coin" from the EMF tech side: what the body actually needs and why these EMFs are causing such havoc for us at a cellular level.

So, I began implementing the things he recommends (all things that reconnect us to the earth and sun) and I could feel my cells healing. Since energy was an emphasis and a passion I had since I was quite young, I found it quite fascinating how the story went "full circle". I used to joke that I was solar powered, but now I have the science to understand that yes, humans actually are solar-powered, and also the science of how and why.

The answer is simple and free: more time in the sun, less time near technology and electricity – but the actual implementation of this brings up questions and often a need for clarification around the details. So, at this point, I am pulling all of this information together into a series of comprehensive courses, from mitigating and managing our EMF environment all the way to understanding the Quantum Biophysics of what is happening and how we can provide what our bodies really need so we can truly heal.

Interesting Side Note: I had injured a nerve in my elbow in September 2019 and it was burning and stinging anytime I went near a magnetic field (produced by flowing electricity). When we started turning our house power off at night while we slept, I was finally able to get some relief from the pain. During the daytime, if near a magnetic field, the pain would return just as sharp and intense as before. This pattern continued for a few months without any change in the degree of pain.

When I was working with Vicki to have her massage out several knotted painful areas, she introduced me to a band that helps support cells affected by radiation. I was skeptical, since there are so many woo-woo (and I'm quite into woo-woo!) things that say they magically shield from EMFs that don't actually help in a measurable way. However, I am also open to finding out experientially, myself.

Note that I haven't ever responded to homeopathics even though my dogs have recovered from some amazing things with them, so I'm pretty clear that the placebo effect isn't likely to work on me.

I also get symptoms from EMFs when I don't

know that there is something near me, sometimes making me more sensitive than my EMF meter!

Within a few days of wearing the band, I noticed the pain in my elbow when near the magnetic fields in the kitchen was less, and then after a few more days, it disappeared altogether. I wasn't able to go in the kitchen at all. Now I can go in there for about a minute and grab something out of the freezer to thaw. This pain did return after shoveling snow and re-injuring that area, but only a week or so later was better again.

The band appears to be some sort of holographic material, and even with my engineering background, I can't quite tell how it works – it does appear to be working at a quantum level on the body to help it deal with these fields better. Based on the metrics that the company has tested, with the Phase Angle (measured through a Body Impedance Meter) increasing, it suggests that the cell membranes are able to hold a charge better, which just so happens to be one of the aims of the neurosurgeon's solution!

It can't block the fields themselves, so it isn't a substitute for cleaning up our EMF environment, but it certainly appears to be able to bring the body some of what it needs to deal with the EMFs we do encounter.

Samantha Vilppu

CHAPTER 8: We've Been Fooled

"Medication, surgery and radiation are the weapons with which conventional medicine foolishly shoots the messengers called symptoms."

Mokokoma Mokhonoana

Commercialization of medicine has its pros and cons. The pros are the advancements in life saving surgeries, transplants and trauma care. Without these lifesaving skills and technology many would prematurely die.

However, medicine today fails miserably in the prevention of diseases and illnesses. Doctors don't get paid to keep you well. The medical industry would go out of business.

Man's notion that he can improve over God's medicine is killing millions of people. It's reported that 250,000 people die every year from medical errors while approximately 128,000 people die annually from properly prescribed, consumed and administered prescription drugs.

It appears that there aren't sufficient clinical studies for new prescription drugs either. Doctors warn their patients of the dangers of using untested drugs.

What?

Sadly, Americans spend more on medicines than all the people of Japan, Germany, France, Italy, Spain, The United Kingdom, Australia, New Zealand, Canada, Mexico, Brazil and Argentina combined.

Medical errors and death from properly prescribed, administered and consumed prescription drugs is the third leading cause of death in the United States following Heart Disease and Cancer. It's not that doctors are practicing "bad medicine". Doctors only know what they are taught in medical school and medical schools are largely funded by the pharmaceutical industry.

Dr. David Classen, associate professor at the University of Utah School of Medicine in Salt Lake City, Utah said, "The system of care is fragmented. Any tools that enable patients to manage their health care needs will be a game changer."

Doctors are taught to treat symptoms with prescription drugs, surgery or referrals out to specialists. Doctors get on average about 6 hours of nutrition in medical school and are not taught natural healing.

Understanding how to work with your body and giving it what it needs to heal itself is one tool that is a game changer and is foundational to knowing what tools you need to heal yourself. This is why I teach muscle testing techniques for you who want God's medicine and can learn how to determine your own needs. Be wise and see your doctor for serious health problems but participate in your own healing.

Your needs could be specific nutritional supplements for hormonal, immune and emotional support. There are times when your muscles, joints, nerves and joints need adjustments with bodywork and chiropractic support. Cognitive (brain) function can be greatly improved with nutrition, laughter, breath work and detoxing. Energy healing works directly by releasing emotional traumas, rebalancing energy and reprogramming thoughts, beliefs, and perceptions.

Society today teaches us to rely on others for our health, wellness and sustenance. As a whole we rely on mechanical devices to cure us, compromised food sources to nourish our malnourished bodies and toxic prescription drugs to stop pain and work its temporary "magic". Often these drugs become addictive and lead to other problems.

Our answers to our health lie within us, hidden in plain sight. Our symptoms are our body's way of communicating what they need and don't need. For instance, excess gas and acid reflux typically is a sign of indigestion. This could stem from an imbalance in gut bacteria caused by the use of antibiotics, sugar, poor diet of junk food and the consumption of grains and high glycemic fruits and vegetables.

Food cravings are a way our body tells us it's not getting the nourishment it needs. This can come from food choices, food allergies, disruption to gut bacterias and also indigestion. Our bodies will crave what it needs.

Depression and anxiety are displaced dis-organized energy in the form of perceptions of thoughts, regrets, traumas, anguish and unresolved emotions.

You have the power to change what you don't like. You have the power with your own mind shift to totally break these chains and set yourself free. This is what I did for me with help from others and you are hardwired with the same God-given power. You might simply need assistance from time to time.

The late Venice Bloodworth, PhD in psychology, explains a universal principle:

"The method is always the same, regardless of what is to be accomplished. First, the idea. Second, visualizing the idea. Third, manifesting the idea. First we make a decision; then, we use the marvelous function of the mind, the imagination, which I call the workshop of the mind, to visualize this change. Since it is a law that energy follows thought, then when the thoughts are flowing in a positive manner, we get positive results."

Modern medicine teaches the use of psychotropic drugs which are addictive, mind altering, toxic and foreign to what your body recognizes it needs to heal itself. I'm taught the opposite. I'm taught to understand the holistic needs of your body and what your body naturally is missing and is looking for. I use God's medicine and remedies, nutrition, homeopathy, supplementation, energy healing and bodywork.

As your body tries to adjust to foreign toxic substances, it will notify you that it doesn't like this assault by creating symptoms. Just read the list of possible side effects on the labels on your prescription drugs. Better yet, listen to the commercials on T.V. The volume is louder when promoting the prescription drug and much softer and harder to capture as they rush quickly through possible side effects.

One side effect of Metformin is possible kidney failure. A family member was properly using Metformin as prescribed for his Type 2 Diabetes. All was going well, or so he thought. His doctor took him off of Metformin when a blood test determined that his kidney function plummeted to 30%. At this point he opted to control his blood sugar with food.

He told me that he was stable at 30% and his doctor was happy with 30% and if his doctor is happy with that number then it's good enough for him. Are you kidding me? No, No, No! I begged him to let me help him get back to 100% function, but his doctor reassured him that he was fine.

Well a few years later I got the dreaded phone call from my daughter that he was in kidney failure facing a kidney transplant because now he was at 17% function and scared. He wanted to try the natural supplement that I was recommending.

He wanted to check with his doctor to see if the supplement would interfere with any of his current treatments before starting. His doctor told him that this wouldn't hurt him but that he didn't believe in nutritional supplements and not to waste his money because they don't work and he can get everything he needed from a good diet. Obviously not.

He chose not to listen to that advice and proceeded with my help. Over the next 2 months his doctor had him scheduled with various appointments getting ready for the transplant. My granddaughter was a perfect match and was on standby with one of her kidneys.

In just one week his kidney function was up to 20% and he was encouraged. Over the course of the next few weeks his function dipped back down to 17%

before jumping to 28%. "I'm confused", his doctor told him. "Kidneys don't repair themselves. Keep doing what you're doing. We're taking you off of the transplant list, you're no longer a candidate" his doctor told him.

I'm not saying to suddenly ditch the meds you are currently using or disregard what your doctor is recommending. I'm just saying there are natural nontoxic ways to work with your body that your body is hardwired to receive so that your body's own immune system and natural ability to heal itself will kick in.

When you no longer need the prescription drugs then your doctor will taper or take you off because you no longer need them to manage or regulate your symptoms because your body is healing.

There are numerous natural methods of healing that your body is hardwired to respond to that are simple and basic. Breathwork is another method.

I'm now going to reintroduce you to your breath as a method of calming your nerves, reducing episodes of anxiety and reducing the harmful effects of stress. Most of us, including me, take our breath for granted. We don't have to even think about it, we just breathe, right?

Did you know that your lungs rely on tiny capillaries? Do you take shallow breaths, or do you breathe deep into your Diaphragm? You don't get enough oxygen with shallow breaths? Your diaphragm is a muscle that needs deep breaths for its strengthening exercises in order to contract and expand your lungs.

Breathing deep into your Diaphragm assists your lungs in delivering more life-giving oxygen to your body while synergistically calming your nerves and shutting down the excess release of your stress hormone, Cortisol.

Cortisol is your fight or flight hormone that responds to stress and grief, shuts down digestion, sex drive, thinking and sleep. It gears you up for battle.

Chi (energy) is also regulated through your breath. Breath and grief have an intimate relationship. Suppressing grief and emotions leads to anxiety. Allow yourself to feel the grief and not suppress it.

However, there is a fine line between feeling

grief and damaging your health. I know a gal who cried and stressed a solid month nonstop over the sudden passing of her dad and ended up in a wheelchair with full blown Multiple Sclerosis. Her Cortisol levels were too high for too long.

Be sure to take care of yourself during the grieving process. Take time for self-care, meditation, music, spending time with family and quiet times with your own breath work.

Here's a breathing exercise that's easy for you to learn: Sit comfortably with your back straight and not touching the back of a chair. Inhale to the count of 4; hold to the count of 7; exhale to the count of 8 while expanding your ribs laterally past your arms for 4 rounds then quick breath in and a quick breath out.

Now relax. Be sure to focus your attention on your breath while you are doing this. Feel your breath flowing through each organ and around and in between each organ. Feel your breath rise up along your back and the front of your torso. If this timing is uncomfortable for you to hold this long, then here is a shorter version.

Inhale to the count of 4; hold to the count of 4;

exhale to the count of 4; pause to the count of 4 and then relax. Repeat until the stress, panic or anxiety has dissipated. Listen for inspiration and intuitive thoughts coming in. Some of your "doors" only open from the inside. Breath is a way of accessing that door.

Communication between your gut, your immune system, and your brain is transmitted through the Vagus Nerve which will relax with this breathing exercise. Feel free to play soft music and eliminate distractions.

The exciting news is that most illnesses and diseases are preventable. Yes, you can heal and prevent most illnesses just with a lifestyle change, proper nutrition, and a calm nervous system in spite of environmental toxins, radiation from cell phones and electronics (EMFs), pesticides, chemtrails, compromised food sources and numerous other stressors.

If you have tried everything you're instructed to do by your health care professionals and are just maintaining the same level of illness, not getting well or continuing to get worse and your doctor has no answers, then your missing link could easily be

Epigenetics and or nutrition.

Epigenetics is the study of organisms and the modifications of the physical structure of their genes altered by their environment. Bruce Lipton, a stem cell biologist, and former cellular Biology professor at the University of Wisconsin's School of Medicine dis-covered that stem cells easily alter their genetic expressions (characteristics) based on their environment.

During his stem cell research at Stanford University he discovered that the medium in which stem cells grow determines the attributes of the cells themselves. So, what does this mean to you?

His research led him to determine that emotions, traumas and environment alter genetic expressions (the detectable effect of a gene) of our DNA. He says that we are "skin covered petri dishes" with our blood being the medium and hormones that alter blood chemistry depending on our mood, attitude and emotions. We truly are our own best friend or our own worst enemy depending on our own emotional reactions to outside stimulation.

Epigenetics also includes inheritable gene

expressions that are passed down from each preceding generation. This explains why there are genetic predispositions in families. These predispositions can include mental illness, depression, aggressive behavior and other cognitive functions along with Cancer and other diseases.

The best part about this is we have the power to change what we don't like or want with emotions, thoughts, intentions and healthy food choices. Some may think this is hokey while giving no thought as to how thinking about getting a drink of water sets in motion all actions including reaching for the glass and turning on the water.

Radiation and EMF's also alter our blood chemistry. For years I held my cell phone on my ear to talk. I put it in my shirt pocket or pants pocket for safekeeping when not in use. Until... one day. I woke up feeling good and was looking forward to going to church. The phone rang and I sat for a moment to talk. It wasn't long before my ear got HOT. Red hot!

All of a sudden, I had a heavy all-consuming force come over me and my body felt very heavy. I immediately felt like I needed to throw up. I quickly got off the phone and dashed to the bathroom just in time to hug the toilet. I had dry heaves for a few hours after that.

I was so sick that I just laid back in the recliner and stayed there the rest of the day. I was sick for 3 days. I have never put my cell phone to my ear or in my pocket ever since that day. As I took back I realize that this was the beginning of my noticeable symptoms with EMFs.

I quit exercising when I enrolled in massage school in July of 2012 by simply getting out of the habit. I spent more time sitting and or standing doing treatments and simply wasn't motivated to start working out again. Fast forward to 2019 and I joined Camp Gladiator, a rigorous 1-hour workout that I should have been able to just jump right back into.

I couldn't believe how soft I was. My heart would pound out of my chest, my lungs gasped for air and my muscles felt like they were suffocating. I would break out into a hard sweat after just 10 minutes of exertion. I took the summer off because we worked out outside and the heat would knock me over.

My body just was taking a beating and it didn't

seem like I was getting stronger. I couldn't figure it out. I am healthy. This just didn't make sense, until...a friend wanted me to test out a band that helped my body deal with radiation poisoning. WHAT?

I heard stories about cell phones, tablets, laptops, computers, WIFI, Bluetooth and big screen T.V. 's emitted harmful radiation but I thought I was immune. I didn't feel the effects, or so I thought. As long as I wasn't exerting myself, I felt just fine except for major brain fog in the morning.

A friend of mine asked me to wear this band for a week and give her feedback. After just a half a day I was back at my workout with superhuman strength, endurance, normal breathing and could actually run the entire long lap and not even break a sweat. I was even talking immediately after running. My body felt so light and airy! I felt like I had lost 40 lbs. WHAT?

I normally only did half of the lap and walked half of that with a little sprinting periodically. I had superhuman strength and endurance for that whole week, UNTIL I gave her back the band.

I definitely wanted my own. She ordered me one. It was refreshing to wake up in the morning with clear sharp mental function whereas previously it was noon before I could think clearly. I just thought I was a night person and didn't like mornings.

Well here I was working out after 2 ½ days without the band and my body was screaming obscenities at me again. My heart was pumping hard, too hard. My whole body was suffocating. Even the muscles in my legs couldn't breathe. Well, needless to say, I don't take my band off and I'm back to my superwoman workouts.

I explained this to Samantha Vilppu, who is extra sensitive to radiation and has been studying the effects for years. She explained to me that the radiation from these devices robs the electrons from our blood which makes our blood sticky and slow to flow. This slows delivery of vital nutrients and oxygen to our cells through our capillaries while suffocating our body. Our lungs and heart are impacted the most making it hard to breathe. My legs felt like they were full of lead with 4G. I can't imagine 5G.

In addition to radiation and toxic prescription drugs our cells take a beating from the current polluted industrial environment. Modern agricultural practices, lack of sufficient nutrition and "food like substances" only compound the problems because we cannot get everything, we need from our food today.

Add traumas and injuries to this mix and there's a direct assault on your health. Your body works 24/7 trying to keep you healthy. It only asks for some support and TLC.

In spite of all the bombardments from the environment, you still have the power to prevent illness, heal yourself and live a healthy happy life. My course material will cover many proactive methods so that you can get well, stay well and maintain the healthiest possible health.

As Americans we have lost the independence and self-sufficiency of our ancestors for a life of convenience and ease. Or is it a life of ease? We live in a hustle and bustle society that stresses over the soaring cost of living, job insecurity, debt, pollutants and our relationships. Stress is the #1 underlying "preexisting" condition for compromised health.

We traded the simple life on the farm, providing for our own needs, and working from home for life in the big city. What did we really gain? As a society we rely on government programs for financial support to offset the out of control cost of living. Many rely on food stamps, subsidized housing, welfare, medical assistance and government grants for education to prepare for a good job, a job that often leads to stress, exhaustion and broke.

We rely on government-controlled schools to tell us how to think and companies that often pay us just enough to get by. Almost every aspect of our lives today is dependent on others. No wonder we as a whole are disconnected from our own self-care and natural healing.

Today life is also full of "landmines" presenting as stress, poor nutrition, vaccines, emotional and physical traumas, ancestral traumas, industrial injuries, finances, unexpected accidents, unresolved emotions and life in general. Whew! Do you even stand a chance at a healthy happy life?

Yes, you do!

This book is mapped out to empower you through awareness, knowledge, skills and facts based on science and nature to set you on a healing trajectory. Yes, your body is hardwired to heal itself but sometimes just needs help in getting back on track with today's environment and "land mines".

Summary:

Nature and Nature's God has designed a mix of opportunities to give us exciting experiences, opportunities to grow our character, develop our strengths and talents and set us apart from others.

What we do with these experiences also determines our health or lack of health. We truly are more in control of our health than we realize.

Sometimes we just don't know how to assist our body in self-healing, this is why I wrote this book and its workbook companion.

You can get the workbook companion to this book here @ https://bit.ly/HardwiredWorkbook

CHAPTER 9: THE HIDDEN TRUTH ABOUT VACCINES

https://www.youtube.com/watch?v=vH6qQWnnWF0

"There is a good deal of evidence to prove that immunization of children does more harm than any good."

Dr. J. Anthony Morris, former Chief Vaccine Control Officer, U.S. Food and Drug Administration

"The greatest threat of childhood disease lies in the dangerous and ineffectual efforts made to prevent them through mass immunizations."

Dr. R. Mendlesohn, Author and Professor of Pediatrics; How To Raise A Healthy Child In Spite Of Your Doctor

When we were children and were exposed to the German measle virus and other viruses. Our immune system cells got busy producing a protective protein antibody to protect us from any future attacks by that particular virus. These antibodies made sure that we have lifetime immunity that is now part of our DNA. Today kids get temporary immunity along with vaccine injuries that come with a different set of side effects that are far more damaging than the virus itself.

Listed on the vaccine labels are possible side effects such as Autism, cancers, ALS, M.S., other Autoimmune diseases and SIDS.

I vividly remember as a very young child getting the German measles, aka Rubella. I couldn't have been much more than 3 years old. Back in the 1950's the doctors had us stay in a dark room while our bodies responded to this virus and our immune systems-built antibodies while fighting off the virus. My mother put blankets over the windows in my room to shut out all the light. Four days seemed like a very long time.

My mother explained to me that as long as I had the German measles I had to stay in the dark because sunlight would make me go blind. I didn't want to lose my sight, so I never even fussed about staying in the dark until the measles were gone. Today we know that we won't go blind in sunlight with this virus.

My mother would knock on my bedroom door,

"Vicki, cover your eyes baby. I'm going to open the door and bring you some food and milk," she announced. I was very obedient and put my head under the covers until she let me know that I could pop my head out.

We sat there in the dark as I sat up in my bed and ate. This was kinda like having a tea party in the dark. "How much longer do I have to stay in here?", I asked. "Just a few more days honey," she reassured me.

Because I was fortunate enough to get the Rubella virus. I have a lifetime immunity because my immune cells got busy and created antibodies that are part of my DNA now and give me full protection like a standing army. Those who receive a vaccine do not have the same protection. Boosters are routinely required. The military loads our soldiers up with an alarming amount of vaccines since there's a limited amount of protection.

One study revealed that getting the Rubella vaccine (MMR) gave the participants anywhere from 39% - 80% protection and a chance of Autism.

My friend Tasha shared a Post on Facebook from

a friend who gathered the list of ingredients that are used to make vaccines and then called Poison Control to see if these were ok to give her child. Here's how the conversation went:

"I gathered all vaccine ingredients into a list and contacted Poison Control. After intros and such, and asking to speak with someone tenured and knowledgeable, this is the gist of that conversation.

Me: *My question to you is how are these ingredients categorized? As benign or poison? (I ran a few ingredients, formaldehyde, Tween 80, mercury, aluminum, phenoxyethanol, potassium phosphate, sodium phosphate, sorbitol, etc.)*

He: *Well, that's quite a list... But I'd have to easily say that they're all toxic to humans... Used in fertilizers... Pesticides... To stop the heart... To preserve a dead body... They're registered with us in different categories, but pretty much poisons. Why?*

Me: *If I were deliberately to feed or inject my child with these ingredients often, as a schedule, obviously I'd put my daughter in harm's way... But what would legally happen to me?*

He: *Odd question... But you'd likely be charged with criminal negligence... perhaps with intent to kill... and of course child abuse... Your child would be taken away from you... Do you know of someone who's doing this to their child? This is criminal...*

Me: *An industry... These are the ingredients used in* *vaccines... With binding agents to make sure the body won't flush these out... To keep the antibody levels up indefinitely...*

He*: <u>WHAT?!</u>*

Tasha also provides a list of questions that you can ask your pediatrician. Since she and at least one of her children were vaccine injured, she took a deep dive into ingredients and side effects.

Here's a list of her questions you can ask your doctor if you are concerned about vaccines:

1, What are 10 ingredients in vaccines other than the viruses themselves?

(Aborted fetal tissue, polysorbate 80, MSG, aluminum, formaldehyde, bovine cells, thimerosal, canine cells, lactose, Phenoxyethanol)

2, Which vaccine ingredient opens the blood brain barrier allowing toxins to enter the brain?

(Polysorbate 80)

3, Which vaccines contain either human aborted fetal tissue, canine cells, monkey cells, chicken cells?

(All)

4, Which vaccines contain neurotoxins such as aluminum or mercury?

(Most)

5, Which vaccines contain carcinogenic ingredients?

(Most)

6, Which vaccines have not been tested on pregnant women yet are recommended by doctors?

(TDaP & Flu)

7, Which vaccines are known to cause either anxiety disorders, anorexia, developmental disorders, autism, seizure disorders, Crohn's disease, diabetes, SIDS...per scientific peer reviewed studies?

(All)

8, Who is Dr. William Thompson and what role does he play at the CDC?

(Senior Lead scientist at the CDC, turned whistleblower)

9, Which vaccines contain live viruses which infect the recipient and can shed to others?

(MMR, Varicella and Rotavirus) Also flu mist which has been recently reintroduced is a live virus and sheds. Additionally, the Dtap/Tdap and Polio vaccines that are NOT live have been shown to cause the vaccinated to become asymptomatic carriers whenever exposed, thus the vaccinated can be spreading the illness, without knowing, at any time.

10, Which country is having dozens of outbreaks in highly vaccinated communities?

(US)

11, Which vaccine is causing an outbreak by the tens of thousands in India and Africa?

(Polio)

12, Which vaccine is routinely given *after* an injury despite it being a preventative vaccine?

(Tetanus/DTaP)

13, What are the various cancer-causing ingredients in vaccines?

(MSG, formaldehyde, Phenoxyethanol)

14, What is the 1986 vaccine Injury act?

(Removes liability from vaccine manufacturers, using taxpayer money to pay for Injury reimbursement IF awarded)

15, How many billions of $$ has the United States vaccine injury court system paid out?

($3.9 billion and counting)

16, Does acquiring mild childhood illnesses such as measles and chickenpox have any long-term health benefits?

(Strengthens the immune system to fight future illnesses like cancer)

17, Which renowned Children's Hospitals have notified recently vaccinated individuals to not visit patients with autoimmune disorders?

(St. Johns and St.Judes also all nicu's)

18, Where is there proof of vaccine induced herd immunity?

(There isn't)

19, Which virus in a vaccine is being manufactured into a cure for cancer?

(Measles)

20, Why is it a horrible idea to give Tylenol before or after vaccines?

(it suppresses the immune system and depletes glutathione which is needed for detoxification)

21, How many milligrams of aluminum make up to 75 doses of vaccines given to children under 18 years old?

(Wayyy more than is considered safe per FDA)

22, Which vaccine given the day of a child's birth contains dangerous levels of aluminum?

(Hep C)

23, Which industrialized country has one of the highest, if not the highest, infant mortality rates as well as vaccine rates?

(US)

24, Which vaccine was given to 40 million Americans and was later revealed to contain a cancer-causing monkey virus?

(Polio)

25, *Which industrialized country has the fanciest hospitals, highest rate of cancer in children, highest rate of children with autoimmune disorders, and most profitable pharmaceutical industry in the world?*

(US)

26, *Which vaccine was involved in the recent CDC whistleblower scandal showing a link to autism and the CDC covered it up?*

(MMR)

27, *Which states in the US require children to maintain the CDC vaccine schedule in order to attend school?*

(California, West Virginia, New York and Mississippi)

28, *What is wrong with natural immunity?*

(It reduces profit of the pharmaceutical industry)

Those who receive vaccines run the risk of possible side effects listed on the individual labels such as: Cancers, ALS, SIDS, Autism, Seizures, Allergies - including food allergies, MS and other Autoimmune diseases. Vaccine manufacturers created thousands of Polio cases when there were very few if any known cases in an attempt to prevent this disease.

Summary:

Vaccines do more harm than the virus they are designed to provide protection from. Man thinks he can improve over God's method of protection.

The debilitating toxins and chemicals in vaccines penetrate the blood brain barrier that God has in place to protect you and your children from heavy metals and toxins.

Robert F. Kennedy Jr. also has case studies and more information on his website: https://childrenshealthdefense.org/news/truth-with-robert-f-kennedy-jr/

If your child is vaccine injured there is a chance of getting compensation from the National Vaccine Injury Compensation Program.

https://www.mctlaw.com/vaccine-injury/

Contact me as well for natural remedies to restore your child's health. There are homeopathy and other natural protocols designed to reverse these injuries.

You can grab my workbook companion here @ https://bit.ly/HardwiredWorkbook

About the Author

What sets Vicki apart from other therapists in her field is her unique ability to see inside her clients and connect energy to energy and see the imbalances and draw on multiple modalities to assist them in healing themselves.

Hardwired to Heal is all about your power to heal yourself.

Vicki Ariatti was born in Mobile, Alabama in December 1951 to parents who had emotional issues and needed more parenting themselves.

As a byproduct of her childhood, Vicki grew up struggling to find her identity and place in society as a productive healthy member.

When she was 8 years old she vowed that when she grew up that she would end child abuse and neglect not knowing how to make that happen.

She continued in her self defeating behaviors and childhood patterns of learning the hard way with trial and errors until later in life when she finally turned her life over to her Heavenly Father for His will and guidance.

Little did she know that the first child she would save as an adult would be her own. Years of healing and transformation have formed the foundation of her career today.

Her clients experience renewed hope and healing when conventional medicine leaves them stuck in chronic pain and dis-ease.

www.ingramcontent.com/pod-product-compliance
Lightning Source LLC
Chambersburg PA
CBHW031210270326
41931CB00006B/501